Second Edition

Edited by

Helane S Fronek MD FACP FACPh

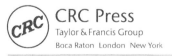

CRC Press
Taylor & Francis Group
Boca Raton London New York

CRC Press is an imprint of the
Taylor & Francis Group, an **informa** business

Published by the Royal Society of Medicine Press Ltd
1 Wimpole Street, London W1G 0AE, UK
Tel: +44 (0)20 7290 2921
Fax: +44 (0)20 7290 2929
Email: publishing@rsm.ac.uk
Website: www.rsmpress.co.uk

Medicine is an ever-changing science. As new research and clinical experience broaden our knowledge, changes in treatment and drug therapy are required. The authors and the publisher of this work have checked with sources believed to be reliable in their effort to provide information that is complete and generally in accord with the standards accepted at the time of publication. However, in view of the possibility of human error or changes in medical sciences, neither the authors nor the publisher nor any other party who has been involved in the preparation or publication of this work warrants that the information contained herein is in every respect accurate or complete, and they disclaim all responsibility for any errors or omissions or for the results obtained from use of the information contained in this work. Readers are encouraged to confirm the information contained herein with other sources. For example and in particular, readers are advised to check the product information sheet included in the package of each drug they plan to administer to be certain that the information contained in this work is accurate and that changes have not been made in the recommended dose or in the contraindications for administration. This recommendation is of particular importance in connection with new or infrequently used drugs.

The right of Helane S Fronek to be identified as editor of this work has been asserted by her in accordance with the Copyright, Designs and Patents Act, 1988.

British Library Cataloguing in Publication Data
A catalogue record for this book is available from the British Library

ISBN-13 978-1-85315-774-5

John J Bergan MD FACS FACPh FRCS Hon(Eng)
Chapters 1 and 11

Jeffrey Buckman MD FACPh
Chapter 17

Craig F Feied MD FACEP FAAEM FACPh
Chapters 1, 5, and 15

Mark D Forrestal MD FACPh
Chapters 5 and 17

Helane S Fronek MD FACP FACPh
Chapters 2, 3, 4, and 16

Mitchel P Goldman MD FACPh
Chapters 8 and 9

Alan H Kanter MD FACPh
Chapter 7

Robert F Merchant MD FACS FACPh
Chapter 10

John Mauriello MD FACPh
Chapter 13

Robert J Min MD MBA FACPh FSIR
Chapter 10

Nick Morrison MD FACS FACPh
Chapters 7, 10, 11 and 12

Diana L Neuhardt RVT
Chapter 2

Jerry G Ninia MD FACOG FACPh
Chapter 15

José-Antonio Olivencia MD FICS FACA FACPh
Chapter 12

Pauline Raymond-Martimbeau MD FACPh
Chapter 2

Neil S Sadick MD FACP FAACS FACPh
Chapters 6 and 9

Robert A Weiss MD FACPh
Chapters 9 and 10

Steven E Zimmet MD FACPh
Chapters 8 and 14

The 21st century has opened the door to a better understanding of the pathophysiology of venous disease based on Doppler duplex findings of the late 20th century.

Now, exploitation of that knowledge is the promise of the future. Not only are the hemodynamic derangements of venous dysfunction better understood, but also the cellular mechanisms of injury in chronic venous insufficiency are being uncovered. Just as minimal invasion has come to general surgery, so has minimal invasion arrived at the treatment of venous disorders. Radiofrequency or laser thermal ablation and chemical ablation with sclerosant foam have been applied with increasing success as a means of taking dysfunctional veins out of the circulation. A greater number of patients with venous disease are being cared for by an increasing number of physicians who have mastered these new technologies. Especially in underdeveloped countries, sclerosant foam is being used in the treatment of venous leg ulcers and even huge varicose veins. Physicians (and their patients, too) are finding that this method of delivering care is effective and affordable. More importantly, wider application of the principles contained in this volume will provide definitive therapy for a group of patients who, in the recent past, have been relegated to supportive or even no treatment because of the belief that they were afflicted with a chronic, unyielding disease.

And so the saga spins on, and as it does so, this book spreads knowledge and betters care. That is the fervent desire of each of the authors of the following chapters. I join them in their desire to make the best care of venous disorders the general rule and not the exception reserved for a very few.

JOHN BERGAN MD
La Jolla, CA

The American College of Phlebology was formed some years ago by a small group of physicians with diverse specialty interests. They had one important thing in common – an interest in the care of patients with venous diseases. These physicians agreed that their medical education and training had been lacking in this area and that the medical community at large was unaware of the prevalence of these disorders and the significant impact that they have on the daily lives of afflicted individuals.

Over the years, the American College of Phlebology has grown to nearly 2000 members and has retained a broad scientific base, including physicians from diverse medical backgrounds, scientists, nurses, and ultrasound technologists. With the College's strong history of scientific, educational, and research development and programming, the American Medical Association recently recognized phlebology as a medical specialty. The rapid growth of this specialty has been supported by and has fueled the interest of many corporations, who have partnered with us to form the Foundation of the American College of Phlebology. Together, we remain dedicated to improving the care of patients with venous disorders by promoting research and education in the field of phlebology, the study of venous disorders. It was for this reason that *The Fundamentals of Phlebology: Venous Disease for Clinicians* was originally written, and the same motivation lies behind this second edition. We hope that the information in this manual will be interesting as well as helpful to clinicians, house staff, and medical students, and that medical educational programs at all levels will recognize the need to include these topics in their training and didactic curricula. In turn, we hope that this will further increase our understanding of the patho-physiology and treatment options for all forms of venous disease and that these advances will become more widely available.

Venous disorders are generally not life-threatening, but they affect millions of people in the United States on a daily basis. They not only cause pain, disability, and hundreds of millions of dollars in healthcare costs, but also negatively impact the quality of life in afflicted patients. Fortunately, we now have the ability to treat nearly all affected patients with minimal invasion, little morbidity and a very high expectation of success.

I thank all of the contributing authors whose interesting work is displayed here and all of those active in the field of phlebology whose work has contributed to the impressive growth of this specialty. The Herculean efforts of our recent President, Dr Steven E Zimmet, have placed the American College of Phlebology in a stronger position to create a great impact in this field, guaranteeing that significant advances will continue to be recognized. Special thanks again go to Mr Christopher Freed, whose ever cheerful input and superb computer expertise have made the creation of both the first and second editions so smooth. This project, and all the many activities of the American College of Phlebology, have benefited from the excellent guidance and attention of Mr Bruce Sanders, our Executive Director. Through the dissemination of this volume, we hope that erroneous teachings and archaic treatments can be laid aside, to make way for new understanding, new techniques and new skills that will afford patients with venous disease healthier and more productive lives.

HELANE S FRONEK MD

The peripheral venous system functions both as a reservoir to hold extra blood and as a conduit to return blood from the periphery to the heart and lungs. Unlike arteries, which possess three well-defined layers, most veins are composed of a single tissue layer. Only the largest veins possess internal elastic membranes, and at best this layer is thin and unevenly distributed, providing little buttress against high internal pressures. The correct functioning of the venous system depends on a complex series of valves and pumps that are individually frail and prone to malfunction, yet the system as a whole performs remarkably well under extremely adverse conditions.

The entire cardiac output volume of 10 L/min is received into end-capillary venules for eventual delivery back to the heart and lungs. A large part of this volume passes into the peripheral venous system of the extremities, where it is received against a reverse pressure gradient, then is passed (mostly) uphill against gravity, against fluctuating thoracoabdominal pressures, and sometimes in the face of additional back pressures such as the elevated right atrial pressures of congestive heart failure. All of this return circulation occurs with no obvious motive force. Considered in this light, the venous system seems almost magical in its function.

Primary collecting veins of the lower extremity are passive, thin-walled reservoirs that are tremendously distensible. Most are suprafascial, surrounded by loosely bound alveolar and fatty tissue that is easily displaced. These suprafascial collecting veins can dilate to accommodate large volumes of blood with little increase in back pressure, so that the volume of blood sequestered within the venous system at any moment can vary by a factor of two or more without interfering with the normal function of the veins. Suprafascial collecting veins belong to the superficial venous system. Outflow from collecting veins is via secondary, or conduit, veins that have thicker walls and are less distensible. Most of these veins are subfascial and are surrounded by tissues that are dense and tightly bound. These subfascial veins belong to the deep venous system.

The superficial venous system

The superficial venous system is a tremendously complicated and extremely variable weblike network of interconnecting veins, most of which are unnamed. A few larger superficial veins are fairly constant in location. Like the deep veins, these superficial veins serve as a conduit to pass blood centrally and eventually into the deep venous system.

The principal named superficial veins of the lower extremity are the small saphenous vein (SSV), which usually runs from ankle to knee, and the great saphenous vein (GSV), which usually runs from ankle to groin.

The small saphenous vein (Figure 1.1)

The small saphenous vein originates in the lateral foot. It passes posteriorly lateral to the Achilles tendon in the lower

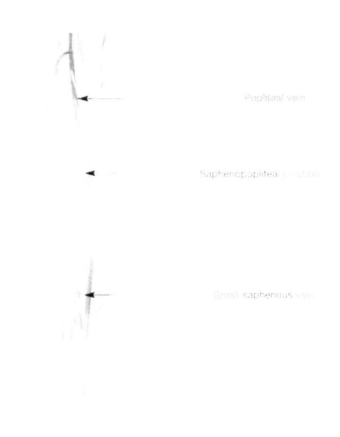

Popliteal vein

Saphenopopliteal junction

Small saphenous vein

Anatomy of the small saphenous vein. Illustration by Linda S Nye)

calf. The SSV usually lies directly superficial to the deep fascia in the midline as it reaches the upper calf, where it enters the popliteal space between the two heads of the gastrocnemius muscles. In two-thirds of cases, it joins the popliteal vein above the knee joint, and in one third of cases, it joins with other veins (most often the GSV or the deep muscular veins of the thigh). In some patients, the SSV may have two or three different termination sites.

The great saphenous vein (Figure 1.2)

The GSV originates in the medial foot and passes anterior to the medial malleolus, then crosses the medial tibia in a posterior direction to ascend medially across the knee. Above the knee, it continues anteromedially, superficial to the deep fascia, and passes through the foramen ovale to join the common femoral vein at the groin crease at a site termed the saphenofemoral junction (SFJ). Large tributaries of the GSV are easily mistaken for the main trunk. Most patients have at least two major tributaries below the knee (the anterior and posterior tributaries, the latter known as the posterior arch vein) and at least two above the knee (the anterior circumflex and posterior circumflex tributaries). These veins usually drain into the GSV distal to the SFJ; however, they may also have a direct connection to the femoral vein. In addition to these veins, there are three pelvic veins that commonly drain into the GSV at the SFJ: the superficial inferior epigastric, the superficial external pudendal, and the superficial circumflex iliac veins. Many patients have a duplicated main GSV trunk in the thigh and some may have three or even four veins, known as anterior or posterior accessory veins, which parallel the main GSV trunk and either reconnect with it usually just above or below the knee or traverse more superficially in the distal thigh.

Perforating veins

Many superficial collecting veins deliver their blood into the great and small saphenous veins, which deliver most of their blood into the deep system through the SFJ and the saphenopopliteal junction (SPJ). However, the SPJ and SFJ are not the only pathways from the superficial system to the deep system. Superficial veins are also connected to a variable number of perforating veins that pass through openings in the deep fascia to join directly with the deep veins of the calf or thigh. Perforating veins usually contain venous valves that prevent reflux of blood from the deep veins into the superficial system. A few named perforating veins are fairly constant in location and are named only as vague groupings. The old nomenclature included Hunter's perforator in the mid thigh, Dodd's perforator in the distal thigh, Boyd's perforator at the knee, and Cockett's perforators in the distal medial calf and ankle and is demonstrated in Figure 1.3. The current nomenclature is noted in Table 1.1.

Saphenofemoral junction

Great saphenous vein

Anatomy of the great saphenous vein. (Illustration by Linda G Nye)

Perforating veins (PV) of the leg	
Foot perforators	Dorsal foot or intercapitular PV Medial, lateral, plantar foot PV
Ankle perforators	Medial ankle, lateral ankle, anterior ankle PV
Leg (calf) perforators	Paratibial, posterior tibial PV (formerly Cockett's perforators) Anterior leg, lateral leg PV Posterior leg PV (medial and lateral gastrocnemius, Intergemellar, para-achillean PV)
Knee perforators	Medial knee PV (formerly Boyd's perforator) Suprapatellar, lateral knee, infrapatellar, popliteal fossa PV
Thigh perforators	Medial thigh PV (formerly Hunter's perforator) (PV of the femoral canal or inguinal PV) Anterior thigh, lateral thigh PV Posterior thigh PV (posteromedial, sciatic, posterolateral PV) Pudendal PV
Gluteal perforators	Superior gluteal, midgluteal, lower gluteal PV

Hunterian perforator

Dodd's perforator

Boyd's perforator

Cockett's perforators

Major named perforating veins of the leg. Illustration by Linda S. Nye.

The deep venous system (Figure 1.4)

All venous blood is eventually received by the deep venous system from which it is returned back to the right atrium of the heart. In most texts the deep venous system is named members of the deep venous system: these below and their above the knee. The principal deep venous route of the leg is called the popliteal vein as it runs above the knee, until it turns upward and anteriorly through the adductor canal in the distal thigh, where it is called the femoral vein (FV) for the remainder of its course in the thigh. Although historically called the "superficial femoral vein," this deep vein should be referred to simply as the femoral vein in order to clarify its position within the deep venous system.

Deep veins of the calf

In the lower leg, three paired axial veins course the anterior tibial vein (ATV), draining the dorsum of the foot; the posterior tibial vein (PTV), draining the medial surface of the foot; and the peroneal vein, draining the lateral surface of the foot. From the ankle, the anterior tibial vein passes upward anterolateral to the interosseous membrane, the posterior tibial vein passes upward posteromedially beneath the medial edge of the tibia, and the peroneal vein passes upward posteriorly through the calf. Venous sinusoids within the calf muscle coalesce to form soleal and gastrocnemius intramuscular venous plexus which drain the peroneal vein is most. In most patients, each

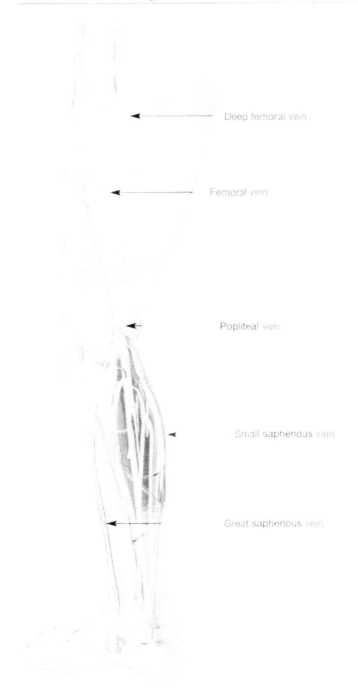

Deep femoral vein

Femoral vein

Popliteal vein

Small saphenous vein

Great saphenous vein

The deep venous system of the leg. (Illustration by Linda S Nye)

one of these is actually a pair of veins flanking an artery of the same name; thus, there are actually six named deep veins below the knee in a typical patient. Just below the knee, the four anterior and posterior tibial veins join with the two peroneal veins to become the single large popliteal vein.

Deep veins of the thigh

The popliteal vein courses proximally behind the knee and then passes anteromedially in the distal thigh through the adductor canal, at which point it is called the FV. The PV and the FV are one and the same, and this is the largest and longest deep vein of the lower extremity. The deep femoral vein (DFV) is a short, stubby vein that usually has its origin in terminal muscle tributaries within the deep muscles of the lateral thigh, but may communicate with the popliteal vein in up to 10% of patients. In the proximal thigh, the FV and the DFV join together to form the common femoral vein (CFV), which passes upward above the groin crease to become the iliac vein.

The calf muscle pump

The passage of blood upward from the feet against gravity depends on a complex array of valves and pumps. Muscle pumps of the calf and foot provide the motive force for venous return. This is frequently called the calf muscle pump or musculovenous pump and is thought to function as the peripheral heart. The calf muscle pump is easy to understand by simple analogy to the common hand-pump bulb of a sphygmomanometer. Before pumping starts, the pressure is neutral and equal everywhere throughout the system. When the hand bulb is squeezed, the intake valve is forced closed and the outflow valve is forced open. Air is pumped into the cuff at high pressure. When the hand bulb is allowed to relax, the bulb re-expands. The inflow valve opens to allow refilling of the bulb.

Each segment of the calf muscle pump works in the same way as the hand bulb of the sphygmomanometer. Inflow to a segment of deep vein is through intake valves from perforating veins as well as from the deep vein segment below. Outflow is through an outflow valve to the deep vein segment above. Squeezing of the vein segment occurs when muscle contraction increases the pressure within a fascial muscle compartment. Just like a sphygmomanometer, the calf muscle pump can achieve pumping pressures of several hundred mmHg before valve failure occurs.

Venous dysfunction

Venous dysfunction develops when venous return is impaired for any reason, and can arise from abnormalities within the deep veins, superficial veins, or a combination. It can result from primary muscle pump failure, from venous obstruction (thrombotic or nonthrombotic), or from venous valvular incompetence, which may be segmental or may involve the entire length of the vein. Immediately after ambulation, the normal pressure within the veins of the lower extremity is extremely low. Normal inflow to the lower extremity veins is purely via arterial inflow; the normal venous system will be more or less refilled after 3–5 minutes of standing. When the entire venous system is filled, the valves float open and venous pressure rises to a maximum exactly equal to the height of the standing column of venous blood from right atrium to foot. This condition triggers an urge to move the legs, activating the muscle pumps and emptying the leg veins.

Primary muscle pump failure

If the calf muscle pump does not work (because of muscle wasting, neuromuscular disease, deep fasciotomies, or local vein valve failure within the muscle fascia sheath), venous blood is never effectively pumped out of the distal extremity. The immediate postambulatory venous pressure will be nearly as high as the pressure after prolonged standing. The volume of venous blood that suffuses the extremity and dilutes arterial inflow will be increased. A smaller fraction of the extremity's venous blood will return to the central circulation each minute, and because arterial blood must flow into congested tissues with elevated hydrostatic pressure, the volume of arterial inflow will actually be reduced.

Deep obstruction

Partial obstruction of the deep veins may have little effect on venous outflow, but severe obstruction produces secondary muscle pump failure. In this case, the muscle pump produces an appropriately high outflow pressure with each contraction, but the volume of venous blood pumped out of the calf is reduced because of the reduced diameter of the outflow tract.

Deep incompetence

If outflow tracts are open and the muscle pump is functional but the valves of the deep veins permit reflux (because of primary agenesis, prior thrombosis, direct trauma, or dilatation with secondary valvular failure), venous blood will be pumped out of the calf in normal volumes but extremity refill will include both normal arterial inflow and pathologic venous retrograde flow. The venous pressure immediately after ambulation may be slightly elevated or it may even be normal, but the veins will refill and dilate very quickly. After a person with deep incompetence stands for only a few seconds, the venous pressure will be nearly as high as the maximum reached after prolonged standing. Again, the volume of venous blood that suffuses the extremity and dilutes arterial inflow will be somewhat increased. A smaller fraction of the extremity's venous blood will return to the central circulation each minute, and because arterial blood must flow into congested tissues with elevated hydrostatic pressure, the volume of arterial inflow will again be somewhat reduced.

Perforator incompetence

Under ordinary circumstances, the bulk of venous blood moves strictly from the superficial to the deep system. Failure of the valves of perforating veins can permit a significant volume of blood to flow from deep veins backward into the superficial system, producing local congestion and venous hypertension. More important, perforator incompetence allows the extremely high pressures generated within deep veins by the calf muscle pump to be communicated to the superficial veins, which are not strong enough to tolerate the pressure. This high pressure (even if intermittent and highly localized) can produce excessive venous dilatation and secondary failure of superficial vein valves. This is one of the major mechanisms for the development of superficial venous incompetence and varicose veins.

Superficial incompetence

Superficial venous incompetence is the most common form of venous disease. Retrograde flow through the superficial venous system occurs when venous valves no longer perform their usual function. This can happen for a variety of reasons. Direct injury, superficial phlebitis, or inflammation may cause primary valve failure. Congenitally weak vein walls may dilate under normal pressures to cause secondary valve failure, or congenitally abnormal valves may be incompetent at normal superficial venous pressures. Normal veins and normal valves may become excessively distensible under the influence of progesterone (as in pregnancy). In other cases, superficial venous reflux is the end result of the introduction of high pressures into otherwise normal superficial veins that were intended to function as a low-pressure system. High pressure causes normal superficial veins to dilate so widely that the thin flaps of venous valves simply no longer meet in the midline.

High pressure can enter the superficial veins by failure of key valves at any point of communication between the deep and superficial systems. Two clinical syndromes of high-pressure superficial system disease are recognized: junctional and perforator. Junctional high-pressure disease results from failure of the primary valve at the junction between the GSV and the CFV (the SFJ) or at the junction between the SSV and PV (the SPJ). Vein dilatation in these cases proceeds from proximal to distal, and patients perceive that a large vein is "growing down the leg." Perforator high-pressure disease results from failure of the valves of any perforating vein. The most common sites of primary perforator valve failure are in the mid-proximal thigh and in the proximal calf. If the primary high-pressure entry point is distal, patients experience the initial development of large clusters of veins in the lower leg, with large veins eventually "growing up the leg" toward the groin.

Introduction

The purpose of the clinical phlebology examination is to determine the extent of the patient's disease and to identify the primary sources of reflux. Additional diagnostic studies are then considered and a treatment plan based upon the examination is formulated. In most cases, the underlying problem of venous insufficiency is valvular incompetence, resulting in bidirectional blood flow (reflux). The most frequent form of the disease, termed primary varicose vein disease, originates in the superficial venous system and is caused by a genetic disorder of the venous wall and/or dysfunction of the venous valves. Less common is secondary varicose vein disease, in which reflux originates in the deep venous system. This occurs because of damaged valves from prior thrombosis or trauma, or from congenital absence of valves. After thrombosis in the deep system, the patient may have both reflux and obstruction. The increased pressure in the deep veins due to impeded outflow and/or volume overload may also cause the perforating veins between the deep and superficial systems to become dilated and incompetent. In turn, this allows high pressure blood flow from the deep veins to enter the low pressure superficial system. In this manner, normal unidirectional control of blood flow is lost. Though far less frequent, varicose veins may be associated with reflux through vulvar varices with or without any relation to the reflux in the lower extremities. Patients may also present with varices that originate in the pelvic veins, including the ovarian and uterine veins. All of these potential sites of pathology are considered as the phlebologist evaluates each patient.

Physical examination

During the examination, the patient should be standing, preferably on a platform. The examiner should have clear viewing of the patient from the umbilicus down to the toes. During inspection, one should look for any irregularities in limb circumference, presence of active or healed ulcer, lipodermatosclerosis, and areas of large varicose veins, reticular veins, or spider veins. The presence of scars on the leg may indicate prior surgery or trauma. On the lower leg, bulges may be either local dilatations of incompetent veins or muscle fascia hernias. The latter will disappear completely when the patient dorsiflexes the foot with the heel remaining on the examination platform. On continuous-wave Doppler, these areas are silent. With duplex ultrasound examination, the venous structure is seen in this area.

With the patient facing the examiner and the foot externally rotated, the distribution of the great saphenous vein (GSV) is observed. Varicosities along the medial thigh and leg may be the GSV itself, but are more frequently tributaries. Either an anterior or posterior accessory vein, the anterior or posterior circumflex veins (which can be seen coursing in their named directions if one observes them more distally in the thigh), or other unnamed tributaries. The medial plantar foot region is examined for the presence or absence of telangiectatic veins referred to as 'corona phlebectatica,' an indication of a more chronic and/or severe condition. The skin changes of chronic venous insufficiency are graded according to the classification described by Widmer (Figure 2.1).

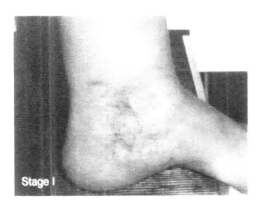 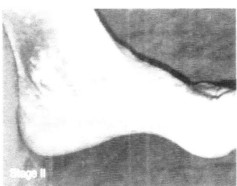 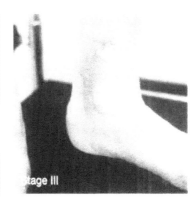

Widmer classification. Images courtesy of Helane S Fronek MD, Robert Stemmer MD, and Walter de Groot MD

Stage I: presence of corona phlebectatica
Stage II: presence of hypo- and/or hyperpigmentation
Stage III: presence of a recent or healed ulcer

The posterior malleolar or posterior arch vein, the posterior tributary of the GSV in the lower leg, is connected to the posterior tibial (Cockett's) perforators. The distal aspect of this vein runs very close to the posterior tibial artery and the phlebologist should be aware of the close proximity of this vessel during sclerotherapy. Occasionally, one may see distended veins overlying an incompetent perforating vein, so-called "blow-out" veins.

As the hands are placed on the medial and lateral thighs, one may detect dilated veins, warmth (which may indicate stagnant or high flow in addition to inflammation), or areas of tenderness. At the knee level, one of the earliest signs of great saphenous insufficiency is the retrocondylar bulge that is felt before it is seen as the great saphenous vein passes behind the medial femoral condyle. Indurated skin and edema may indicate the presence of more severe disease. The presence of hard nodules within varicose veins is frequently due to a prior episode of superficial thrombophlebitis.

When examining the small saphenous vein (SSV), it is best to have the patient facing away from the examiner with the knee slightly flexed. It is easiest to trace the vein from its origin around the lateral malleolus across the Achilles tendon up to the mid calf, where the SSV emerges from the muscular fascia and is often dilated when incompetent. The SSV may also be c ted at the popliteal fossa, and a spongy, tubular vertical structure may be appreciated. Dilated, tortuous calf veins may be the result of incompetence of the GSV, the SSV, or both, and frequently are intersaphenous tributaries that connect the two veins. As in the case of the GSV, since the skin changes due to SSV insufficiency will be seen at the distal portion of the vein, the lateral ankle region should be carefully inspected for the above mentioned skin changes.

The subcutaneous abdominal vein or superficial epigastric vein is one of the three pelvic tributaries that drain into the saphenofemoral junction (SFJ). Insufficiency may result in dilated, tortuous varicosities along the lower abdomen and pubic regions. Insufficiency of this vessel is always abnormal and should alert the phlebologist to possible underlying iliofemoral venous obstruction.

Insufficiency of the external pudendal veins is manifested in approximately 10–15% of patients as dilated varicose or reticular veins in the labia or the proximal medial thigh close to its junction with the pubis. Many times, patients will not complain of these, and it requires an astute examiner to find them. A history of vulvar varicosities during pregnancy or symptoms of heaviness or aching in the labia or pelvis with menses should alert the physician to the likelihood of pudendal insufficiency.

The Doppler device detects frequency shifts from ultrasound waves that are reflected from blood cells coming towards or going away from the Doppler ultrasound probe. The most commonly utilized transducers employ frequencies of 4 MHz, which is a deeper penetrating frequency with a maximum sensitivity 4–4.5 cm from the skin surface, or 8 MHz, which has less penetration and is able to evaluate vessels approximately 0.5–2 cm from the skin surface. It is this higher-frequency probe that is used to evaluate the superficial venous system. The 4 MHz probe is usually used to evaluate the deep system, although it is also useful to have a 4 MHz probe available to evaluate the superficial system in larger patients.

With the patient standing, the probe is placed over the vein in question at an angle to the skin between 30° and 45°, and compression is applied distal to the probe to create a flux (antegrade flow) sound. Due to its unidirectional valves, in a normal vein, there will be no reflux or reversal of flow upon release of the distal compression. If a reflux sound is heard after release of the distal compression, this is abnormal and diagnostic of venous valvular insufficiency. Incompetence of the valves can also be evaluated by means of proximal compression. When compressing proximal to the probe along the course of the vein, there should be no sound or a very short sound of flow until the valves snap shut. When the proximal compression is released, there should be increased flow in the forward direction. In an incompetent vein, with application of proximal compression, there is an immediate reflux sound of increased frequency as the compressed blood column moves towards the probe. It is also possible to utilize the Valsalva maneuver as another method of proximal compression; however, some patients are unable to perform a Valsalva correctly. Also, competent valves proximal to the vein segment being examined will prevent reflux into an incompetent vein.

With the leg externally rotated approximately 40° and slightly flexed and with the foot kept flat and the weight on the contralateral leg, the femoral vein and the GSV can be evaluated. First, the femoral artery is found, and the Doppler transducer is then moved medially until the much louder, spontaneous sound of blood is heard within the femoral vein. The GSV may then be examined beginning just distal to the inguinal crease, and should be checked for reflux at the SFJ, mid-thigh, knee, and calf levels, as it may be incompetent in any or all of these segments.

To find the popliteal vein, the probe is placed in the popliteal fossa, searching for the popliteal artery signal, usually to be found lateral to the midline. The popliteal vein runs in close proximity to the artery, and it is possible to distinguish the venous sound from the arterial one. The Valsalva maneuver is generally not helpful here. The position of the patient for evaluating the SSV is similar to that of the physical examination. The probe can be placed at the popliteal fossa, the inferior aspect of the point where the SSV emerges from the calf, and just lateral to the Achilles tendon in order to hear SSV flow. Although there are several techniques that will help to distinguish the SSV from the popliteal vein, due to the complexity of   anatomic area, continuous-wave Doppler can only be used as a screening evaluation. Duplex ultrasound is necessary to obtain a clear understanding of the anatomy and flow in this region.

Few phlebologists today would dispute the opinion that the single most important advance in the field of phlebology has been the advent of duplex ultrasound imaging. It is only with duplex that we have realized the incredible complexity and variability of the superficial venous system. Given this variability, our ability to see each patient's unique pathology is invaluable as we attempt to restore normal flow within the system. Duplex is now used for diagnosis of both deep and superficial venous disease, prognostic evaluation, pretreatment mapping of the superficial system, intraoperative imaging and guidance, and post-treatment assessment of therapeutic success as well as diagnosis of the reason for treatment failure.

As awareness of the serious consequences of venous disease has grown, considerable effort has been made to improve the available treatment methods, and it is ultrasound technology that has fueled the dramatic advances in treatment options. The diagnostic capabilities of ultrasound continue to progress, and it is likely that ultrasound will continue to play an essential role in phlebology. Thus, the practitioner should obtain an understanding of ultrasound fundamentals and become proficient in scanning and in recognizing the abundant variations in venous anatomy.

Duplex systems bring together a real-time, brightness mode (B-mode) imaging system and a Doppler signal processor into a single, integrated unit. The duplex image created by manipulating the sound waves produces B-mode imaging of the vascular anatomy and surrounding soft tissue (displayed as grayscale pixels), while Doppler imaging provides simultaneous information about the flow events (displayed as a pulsed spectral waveform and/or color flow pixels) within the vessel. Spectral displays demonstrate essentially the same information as audible Doppler. Duplex allows the examiner to measure the flow within each individual vessel, while continuous-wave Doppler samples flow in all vessels within its path, making the interpretation of any obtained signal ambiguous. And, unlike audible Doppler, the information from a duplex evaluation is processed for individual frequency components onto a graph, enabling the skilled examiner to document precise quantification of the disease. Color Doppler hues correspond to Doppler shift frequencies and flow acceleration. Additionally, specific colors are coded to represent direction of flow, permitting immediate identification of any retrograde flow.

Recent design packaging by manufacturers to create ease of use and affordability has downplayed the underlying complexity of ultrasound. Overall design characteristics of the equipment play an extremely important role in the results obtained. However, advanced duplex systems, regardless of size or specific use, require a thorough understanding of the physics and principles of ultrasound to optimize their full diagnostic potential and are not intended for the casual user. Diagnostic quality from ultrasound relies on the proper education of the ultrasonographer, as well as diligent study and practice.

Deep vein examination

Duplex ultrasound has been used since the 1980's to diagnose obstruction in the deep veins, primarily in the lower extremities. Imaging the deep veins requires high-resolution duplex equipment with accompanying linear transducers with imaging frequencies ranging from 4 to 7 MHz and/or from 2 to 5 MHz curvilinear for larger patients or edematous extremities, and is typically performed with the patient supine. Three techniques are utilized to evaluate the deep veins in order to exclude deep vein thrombosis (DVT): compression of the vein, color Doppler, and spectral Doppler. The most reliable of these techniques is compression of the vein from the groin to the ankle. Normal vein walls collapse fully when minimal probe pressure is applied at the skin surface. In principle, only the venous segments that have been compressed can be accurately evaluated. Therefore, multiple transverse (cross-sectional) images are obtained along the full length of the deep veins to include the common femoral, femoral (formerly termed superficial femoral), profunda femoral, popliteal, tibial, peroneal, and anterior tibial veins. When performed correctly, an abnormal compression test (failure to completely collapse the vein with probe pressure) confirms the presence of venous thrombosis. When thrombosis is present, the internal echo characteristics within the vein will appear hyperechoic. Other characteristics of the vein are considered, including diameter in comparison with the adjacent deep artery. Longitudinal images of the deep veins with color duplex are obtained to confirm patency and examine flow hemodynamics. Deep veins sampled with spectral Doppler document flow dynamics that may also be used to support the diagnosis of DVT. Normally, patent veins will demonstrate spontaneous flow phasicity (showing changes with respiration), whereas continuous flow through the entire respiratory cycle is suspicious for venous thrombosis/stenosis. When obstruction is chronic, however, the flow pattern may appear normal because of collateralization. Indeed, the presence of collateral vessels may be interpreted as evidence of old thrombosis.

Reflux of the deep veins can be verified by using spectral and color Doppler, relying on various maneuvers to observe flow in response to valve closure/function. These may include the use of distal or proximal manual vein compression, Valsalva, or a rapid cuff inflation device. Force imposed through the vein creates a pressure gradient causing normal one-way valves to close. Extensive research has established that normal valve function in all veins (excluding the common femoral vein) results in retrograde flow of no greater than 0.5 s. Retrograde flow in the common femoral vein should be no greater than 1.5 s. The extent of reflux necessary to produce clinical symptoms is yet to be discovered. Reflux may be seen on grayscale as the movement of echogenic aggregates of blood cells in the retrograde direction, or with color flow.

Superficial vein examination

Evaluation of the superficial anatomy with duplex ultrasound has suffered from a lack of uniform standardization of techniques, although minimum standards of diagnosis do exist and continue to be developed as the demand for diagnostic duplex studies of the superficial venous system grows. The Union International de Phlébologie (UIP) recently published a consensus document on duplex ultrasound evaluation. Treating the exact source of reflux is the therapeutic goal and therefore precise information regarding the sites of reflux is necessary. The diagnostic duplex study can be extremely accurate in determining the exact sources of reflux.

Imaging the superficial veins requires high-resolution duplex equipment and accompanying linear transducers with imaging frequencies ranging from 7.5 to 13 MHz. Many venous flow problems involve slow-moving blood, and that means low Doppler shift frequencies. Indeed, the frequencies may be below the lowest frequency threshold for the instrument. For example, if the lowest velocity a 7.5 MHz Doppler can depict is 6 cm/s, then slower flow would be missed. Therefore, the highest-frequency transducer and most sensitive Doppler system available should be chosen, as slow-moving blood is the primary target for diagnosis. Slow-moving blood may not register a color shift; therefore, examination in grayscale should be performed when reflux is suspected but not initially observed (Figure 2.2).

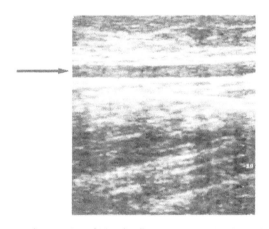

Aggregates of blood cells are seen moving through a vein (arrow) on grayscale. (Image courtesy of Helane S Fronek MD)

The examination is performed with the patient standing, as this will improve accuracy or, at least, standardization. The use of a platform device may maximize comfort for the examiner. Not all the superficial vein networks are formally named, and a thorough understanding of the anatomical landmarks in relation to the superficial veins must be appreciated. The non-weight-bearing extremity is evaluated and should include the GSV, SSV, and large tributaries in multiple locations/segments and in numerous views. The veins are examined from their junction with the deep system (the SFJ for the GSV and the saphenopopliteal junction (SPJ) for the SSV) through their entire course. Both saphenous veins run within fascial compartments, giving rise to the term "saphenous eye" to describe their appearance on ultrasound examination in the transverse view (Figures 2.3 and 2.4).

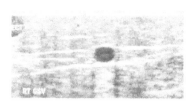

The GSV within a fascial compartment forms a "saphenous eye." (Image courtesy of CompuDiagnostics, Inc., Paradise Valley, AZ)

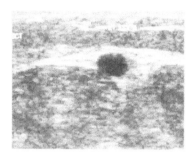

The enlarged SSV seen between the two heads of the gastrocnemius muscle. (Image courtesy of CompuDiagnostics, Inc., Paradise Valley, AZ)

The GSV may be seen to be single or multiple – the duplication of the GSV may continue through the thigh, or one of the trunks may travel more superficially, either parallel to the GSV (anterior or posterior accessory saphenous vein) or it may change its direction to become either the anterior circumflex tributary, the posterior circumflex tributary, or another unnamed tributary. The GSV is normally less than 4 mm in diameter and the SSV is usually less than 3 mm in diameter, although reflux, rather than size, determines abnormality within a vein. The anatomy is best defined with a transverse image, whereas flow is more easily identified and documented in a longitudinal image.

Though not a part of the superficial venous system, perforator veins are included in the examination (Figure 2.5). Perforator veins are noted in the superficial compartment and

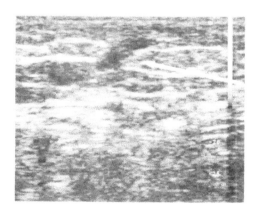

Perforator veins (arrow) pierce the deep fascia to allow normal flow from the superficial venous system to the deep venous system. Bidirectionality of flow within perforator veins is the diagnostic criterion of insufficiency. (Image courtesy of Helane S Fronek MD)

penetrate through the deep fascia to join a deep vein. Perforator vein valves prevent outward flow when functioning properly.

Using duplex ultrasound, retrograde flow can be diagnosed with proper techniques, and must include creating adequate physiologic pressure gradients to demonstrate valvular incompetence. This can be accomplished by compression distal to the probe, followed by release; compression proximal to the probe, followed by release; or by having the patient perform a Valsalva maneuver. Standardization of the compression may be achieved through the use of a rapid cuff inflation/deflation device. Normal valve function should demonstrate retrograde flow no greater than 0.5 s in duration, and the source of reflux must be clearly understood.

While the clinical presentation of superficial thrombophlebitis is evidenced by localized tenderness, erythema, induration, and warmth, and may be confused with cellulitis or other inflammatory conditions, it can also be readily identified with real time imaging. An inability to compress and collapse the walls of the underlying superficial vein by exerting pressure with the transducer confirms the presence of thrombus. Other characteristics of the vein are considered, including the presence of an echogenic mass within the vein lumen. Multiple transverse (cross-sectional) images should be obtained along the vein segment to document the location and extent of the thrombosis. Further evaluation of the deep system is indicated, especially if the proximal GSV is involved, to exclude thrombus extension.

Ultrasound-assisted procedures

Ultrasound imaging allows visualization of the precise location of veins within the superficial compartment, and is an excellent resource to guide treatment of abnormal veins. Innovative, minimally invasive options to ablate the abnormal veins with radiofrequency catheters, laser fibers, and/or sclerotherapy offer patients effective alternatives to invasive vein stripping, and require assistance with ultrasound guidance. A comprehensive knowledge of ultrasound anatomy and instrumentation is imperative to direct the experienced hands of the practitioner.

Ultrasound "mapping" or marking of the skin prior to the procedures identifies the diseased veins to be treated. Ultrasound may then be used to guide needle puncture into the vein, verify placement of guidewires and tumescent anesthesia to confirm proper final location of catheters and/or laser fibers in the venous segment to be treated, and monitor the immediate response to treatment, including venous spasm (Figure ...). The benefit of skilled direct visualization to assist treatment includes reduced risks and complications.

Post-treatment assessment

While it is gratifying to observe success following treatment, many patients do encounter treatment failure. Although treat-

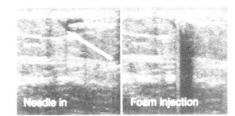

Ultrasound imaging during sclerotherapy using a foamed sclerosant allows visualization of the abnormal vein, placement of the needle within the vein (arrow), movement of the sclerosant, which displays exquisite echogenicity in the foamed state, and spasm of the vessel in response to interaction of the sclerosant with the endothelium. Image courtesy of CompuDiagnostics ... Paradise Valley, AZ)

ment resistance does occur, often the reason stems from previously unrecognized reflux in other areas. Early intervention is key, begins with identification of the site(s) of insufficiency, and may require additional therapy. Interval follow-up will reassure the patient and monitor progress. Post-procedure evaluation is geared toward documenting obliteration of the lumen of the vessel and progressive shrinkage of the diameter with eventual disappearance of the vein. Occlusion of the vein with incompressibility and echogenicity within the lumen can be seen within days after some procedures. Contraction of the vein may not be found for several months after the effective treatment. If the phlebologist notes recurrent varicose veins, persistent pigmentation over a treated vein (lasting longer than 1 year), or persistent symptoms or skin changes, reassessment of the treated vein(s) is indicated.

In addition, since varicose vein recurrence may be due to many factors, including the chronic, progressive nature of varicose vein disease, regular surveillance even after successful treatment is important. The examiner should possess a comprehensive knowledge of expected outcomes and potential complications, including thrombophlebitis and DVT. The previously discussed duplex equipment and operator quality are important factors contributing to the accuracy of measuring the success of treatment.

Functional testing for venous disease

Complete evaluation of the patient with venous disease requires two investigations, one to determine which anatomic sites are involved, and the other to determine what effect these abnormalities have on the function of the venous system. The former component of the evaluation is best accomplished using duplex ultrasound examination, but the significance of the findings will still be uncertain. An analogy may be drawn between the components of a venous evaluation and those required in other medical assessments. In a cardiology patient study, the angiogram will define the anatomic sites of obstruction, while the exercise treadmill test will reveal the functional impairment resulting from these abnormalities. So it is that we may need both anatomic and functional determinations if we wish to truly understand the condition of our patients.

Indications

For many patients with minor degrees of venous abnormality, a functional study will not add to our knowledge; however, there are several situations in which functional evaluation is useful. In patients found to have reflux in both the deep and superficial venous systems, functional testing may help to determine the relative contribution of each system to the patient's problem, and in the setting of deep venous obstruction, it may help to define what role the varicose or saphenous veins play in venous outflow. In patients with large varicose veins, a functional study will indicate if venous hemodynamics have been affected, and, therefore, if treatment is necessary. Patients with venous ulceration and chronic venous insufficiency may benefit from both baseline and post-treatment studies, in order to determine whether a particular therapy has actually improved the venous hemodynamics. Lastly, when patients present with unusual forms of leg pain, a normal functional study will help to rule out venous insufficiency as a contributing factor.

Methods

Photoplethysmography

Photoplethysmography (PPG) is probably the easiest method to incorporate into daily practice, due to its reliability and reproducibility. The test requires a digital photoplethysmograph, a small device that can be easily stored and transported, and it may be performed accurately by an assistant. The test takes approximately 10 minutes to perform.

An infrared light transmitter and sensor are placed on the leg, approximately 10 cm above the medial malleolus. Infrared light is absorbed by hemoglobin; a certain amount of the transmitted light that is not absorbed will be reflected back to the machine. Therefore, with venous congestion, there is more hemoglobin to absorb the light and less can be reflected to the machine. Conversely, after venous outflow, there is less hemoglobin to absorb the light and more may be reflected to the machine.

The exercise portion of the test consists of eight active dorsiflexions followed by a period of rest with the patient in a sitting position. One can evaluate venous outflow as well as reflux. The outflow is visualized by the rise in the curve and the reflux is determined by the time it takes the curve to return to a steady level. In a normal leg, this time, called the venous refilling time (VRT), should be at least 25 s (Figure 2.7). Values less than this indicate the presence of reflux (Figure 2.8).

In a patient with deep and superficial insufficiency, one can repeat the test with a tourniquet compressing the superficial veins either just above or below the knee. If the VRT was initially <25 s and lengthens with placement of the tourniquet, this is indicative of significant superficial reflux. If reflux is suspected in a particular vein, repeating the PPG while applying manual pressure over the specific vein will allow assessment of the effect that treatment of that vein will have on venous hemodynamics (Figure 2.9).

Another use of PPG is to determine the efficiency of the calf muscle pump. This measurement is obtained by performing the "tilt test." First, instead of the patient performing the exercise portion of the test, they lie on their back while their leg is elevated for the same count of eight, and then they assume a sitting position for the refilling portion of the test. Dividing the change in height of the curve (V_0) obtained with 8 dorsiflexions by the V_0 obtained during the tilt test will give a fraction.

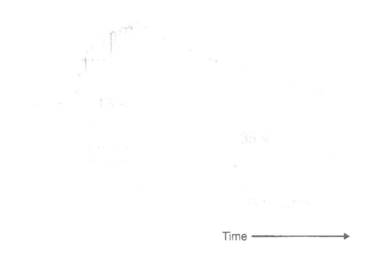

Time ⟶

Normal PPG tracing. (Image courtesy of Hemodynamics, Inc., from brochure for the AV-1000 System)

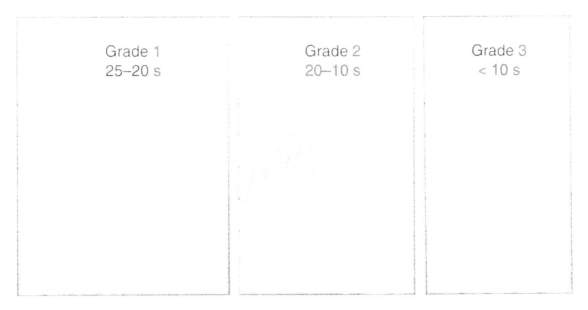

Grade 1	Grade 2	Grade 3
25–20 s	20–10 s	< 10 s

The duration of the venous refilling time can be used to grade the severity of venous insufficiency. (Image courtesy and copyright of Ganzoni & Cie AG SIGVARIS, from Sclerotherapy of Varicose Veins, by Robert Stemmer, 1990)

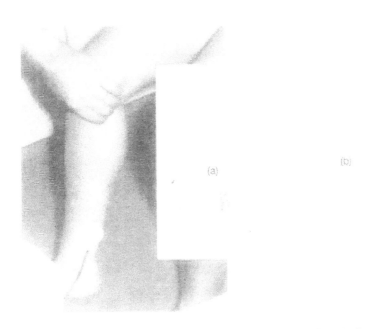

(a) PPG tracing showing abnormally rapid refilling time, indicating significant reflux. (b) The tracing is normalized by compressing the GSV, proving that the etiology of the pathology is GSV insufficiency. (Image courtesy and copyright of Ganzoni & Cie AG SIGVARIS, from Sclerotherapy of varicose veins, by Robert Stemmer, 1990)

When multiplied by 100, this will give an approximation of the ejection fraction of the musculovenous pump.

In using PPG for the evaluation of atypical leg pain, if the clinical examination does not disclose any obvious venous disease, the Doppler test is normal, and the VRT obtained by the PPG is normal, one can generally say that venous insufficiency is not responsible for the leg pain.

Air plethysmography

Air plethysmography (APG) is a more complicated test that is significantly more operator-dependent than digital PPG but it

plus provides additional information regarding the patient's venous status (Figure 2.11):

1. A plastic cuff is placed around the top of patient's calf with the leg elevated on a block and the hip externally rotated with the knee slightly flexed.

2. A small volume of air is injected into the cuff for calibration and then the patient is asked to stand. The change in pressure exerted on the cuff by the distended calf is used to calculate the venous volume (VV) and rapidity of reflux: venous filling index (VFI) = 90% of VV divided by the time it takes to fill 90% of VV (VFI90 = times 10).

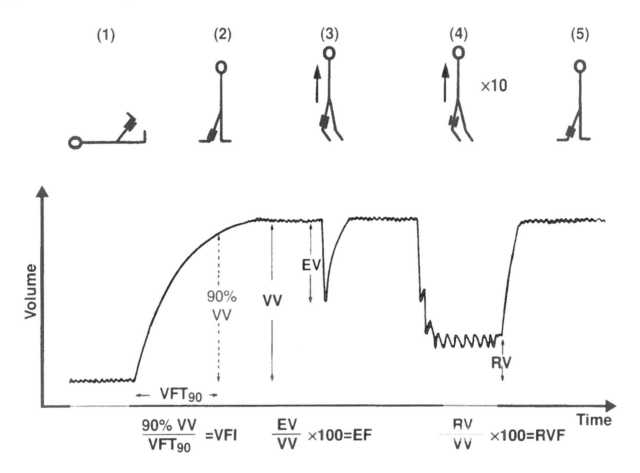

Air plethysmography. (Image courtesy of and reprinted from Journal of Vascular Surgery, V5, Christopoulos, DG. p. 148 copyright 1987, with permission from The Society for Vascular Surgery and The American Association for Vascular Surgery)

3. The patient is then asked to perform one tiptoe motion, in order to measure the volume of blood ejected by the musculovenous pump: ejection fraction (EF) = ejected volume divided by VV, times 100.
4. The patient then performs a further 10 tiptoes.
5. The volume of blood that remains after these additional tiptoes is used to determine the residual volume in the leg, or venous congestion: residual volume fraction (RVF) = residual volume divided by VV, times 100.

An outflow determination, similar to impedance or strain-gauge plethysmography, may be obtained by inflating a cuff around the thigh while the patient is in the initial supine, rotated-hip, and flexed-knee position. This pressure is maintained until a steady state is achieved and then the cuff is rapidly deflated, watching for the outflow from the leg. Rapid outflow generally rules out DVT or chronic obstruction. This test is particularly useful as a noninvasive way of determining if a varicose vein in a patient with a history of DVT or known chronic obstructive disease is functioning as the outflow track, and thus should not be removed or closed. To determine this, one performs the test with manual pressure over the varicose vein. This pressure is maintained for several seconds following cuff deflation. The manual pressure is then removed. If the outflow is at first slow, and after the varicose vein is no longer compressed the outflow becomes more rapid, one can conclude the patient relies on this particular varicose vein for venous outflow.

Previously, phlebograpy (venography) was considered the gold standard for DVT diagnosis, but it is seldom done now. However, it remains a research tool, especially in DVT prophylaxis investigations.

Computed tomography (CT) scans and magnetic resonance imaging (MRI: specifically magnetic resonance venography, MRV), although expensive, are finding broad applications. They are especially applicable in situations of uncertainty such as the clinical suspicion of a pelvic mass, when duplex studies of the leg demonstrate ambiguous results that do not explain the pathology identified on physical examination (e.g., varicosities without apparent duplex-documented reflux source), and suspected pelvic congestion syndrome. CT scans, MRV, and duplex scans reveal information additional to phlebography regarding surrounding tissues, and may establish a differential or definitive diagnosis. When there is pronounced unilateral limb swelling, abnormal spectral Doppler (continuous or high-pitched flow in the common femoral vein) suggestive of proximal obstruction, or if iliac vein thrombosis (May-Thurner syndrome) is otherwise suspected, CT and/or MRV are also indicated. When a vascular malformation is suspected, the evaluation must include lymphatic imaging such as lymphoscintigraphy in addition to CT, magnetic resonance arteriography (MRA), and MRV. Limitations of both CT scans and phlebography are radiation exposure and contrast media complications. These are not present in MRI.

Discussion

Clinical evaluation of the phlebology patient is essential in determining the location and extent of pathology and formulating a treatment plan. Although duplex ultrasound plays a pivotal role in the practice of phlebology, any duplex ultrasound examination should be preceded by a thorough medical history and targeted physical examination, which will direct the attention of the ultrasonographer and enhance the yield of the examination. Functional tests are used infrequently, but have specific indications when particular questions arise. MRI or CT scans may be helpful when considering the diagnosis of pelvic vein disease and vascular malformations, or when the previous evaluation has not yielded a definitive diagnosis. The completed examination should result in a systematic approach to diagnosis and treatment. Clearly, the complexity of venous disease is not to be taken lightly. For this reason, an accurate preliminary evaluation of each phlebology patient, including duplex ultrasound examination, will contribute to the best outcome in each situation.

Bibliography

Bradbury A, Evans C, Allan P, et al. What are the symptoms of varicose veins? Edinburgh Vein Study cross sectional population survey. BMJ 1999; 318: 353-6.

Bygdeman S, Aschberg S, Hindmarsh T. Venous plethysmography in the diagnosis of chronic venous insufficiency. Acta Chir Scand 1971; 137: 423-8.

Christopoulos D, Nicolaides AN. Air plethysmography in the assessment of the calf muscle pump in man. J Phlebol 1986; 1:35-42.

Coleridge-Smith P, Labropoulos N, Partsch H, et al. Duplex Ultrasound Investigation of the Veins in Chronic Venous Disease of the Lower Limbs - UIP Consensus Document. Part I. Basic Principles. Eur J Vasc Endovasc Surg 2006; 31: 83-92.

Darke SG, Vetrivel S, Foy DMA, et al. A comparison of duplex scanning and continuous wave Doppler in the assessment of primary and uncomplicated varicose veins. Eur J Vasc Endovasc Surg 1997; 14: 457-61.

Goldman MP, Bergan JJ, Guex JJ. Clinical methods for sclerotherapy of varicose veins. In. Sclerotherapy: Treatment of Varicose and Telangiectatic Leg Veins, 4th edn. St Louis, MO: Mosby, 2007. Chap 19.

Grondin L, Raymond-Martimbeau P. Superficial venous disease. In. Leclerc JR, ed. Venous Thrombo-embolic Disorders. Philadelphia, Lea & Febiger, 1991: 412-33.

Grouden MC, Stanley ST, Colgan MP, et al. Duplex imaging of the sapheno-femoral junction is the test of choice in patients with primary varicose veins. J Vasc Technol 1993; 17: 71-3.

Guex JJ, Hiltbrand B, Bayon JM, et al. Anatomical patterns in varicose vein disease. Phlebology 1995; 10: 94-7.

Hofer M. Teaching Manual of Color Duplex Sonography. New York: Thieme, 2001: 8-16, 77-84.

Kerner J, Schultz-Ehrenburg U. Functional meaning of different injection tests in the course of sclerotherapy. Phlebology 1989; 4: 123-31.

Killewich LA, Martin R, Cramer M, et al. An objective assessment of the physiologic changes in the postthrombotic syndrome. Arch Surg 1985; 120: 424-6.

Knight RM, Vin F, Zygmunt JA. Ultrasonic guidance of injections into the superficial venous system. In. Davy A, Stemmer R, eds. Proceedings of the XIth World Meeting of the Union Internationale de Phlébologie, London, 1989. Montrouge: John Libbey Eurotext, 1989.

Mantoni S, Hasbarra V, Danielsson G, et al. Endovenous management of saphenous vein reflux. Presented at the American Venous Forum, Dana Point, CA. February 18-21, 1999.

Masuda EM. Prospective study of duplex scanning for venous reflux: comparison of Valsalva and pneumatic cuff techniques in the reverse Trendelenburg and standing positions. J Vasc Surg 1994; 20: 711-20.

McKeon LC, Bergan JJ. Venous reflux examination: technique using miniaturized ultrasound scanning. J Vasc Technol 2001; 25: 149-66.

Myers KA, Ziegenbein RW, Zeng GH, Matthews PG. Duplex ultrasonography scanning for chronic venous disease: patterns of venous reflux. J Vasc Surg 1995; 21: 605-12.

Nix ML, Troillett RD. The use of color in venous duplex examination. J Vasc Technol 1991; 15: 123-8.

Pearce WH, Ricco JB, Queral LA, et al. Hemodynamic assessment of venous problems. Surgery 1983; 93: 715-21.

Petros RL, Schwartz RA. Practical Doppler Ultrasound for the Clinician. New York: Williams & Wilkins, 1992: 11-18, 69-133-8.

Raymond-Martimbeau P. The role of duplex ultrasound in the sclerotherapy of varicose veins. Phlebology Digest 1994; 7: 4-9.

Raymond-Martimbeau, P. Ultrasound imaging and color flow Doppler of the superficial venous system. In. Davy A, Stemmer R, eds. Proceedings of the XIth World Meeting of the Union Internationale de Phlébologie, London, 1989. Montrouge: John Libbey Eurotext, 1989: 367.

Raymond-Martimbeau, P. Duplex ultrasonography assessment of anatomical variations as a guide to sclerotherapy. In. Raymond-Martimbeau P, ed. Phlebologia. Houston, TX: Dallas PRM Editions, 1991: 48-52.

Raymond-Martimbeau, P. Echographie endovasculaire. J Mal Vasc 1992; 17: 135-8.

Raymond-Martimbeau, P. Echographie endo-veineuse. Phlebologie 1991; 44: 629-39.

Raymond-Martimbeau P. Intravenous ultrasound: a new technology for venous assessment. In. Raymond-Martimbeau P, ed. Phlebologia. Houston TX: Dallas PRM Editions, 1991: 53-9.

Sandager G, Williams LR, McCarthy WR, Flinn WR, Yao JST. Assessment of venous valve function by duplex scan. Braz J Med 1986; 10: 626-9.

- van Bemmelen PS, Bedford G, Beach K, Strandness DE. Quantitative segmental evaluation of venous valvular reflux with duplex ultrasound scanning. J Vasc Surg 1989; 10: 425–31.
- van Bemmelen PS, Mattos MA, Hodgson KJ, et al. Does air plethysmography correlate with duplex scanning in patients with chronic venous insufficiency? J Vasc Surg 1993; 18: 796–807.
- Vasdekis SN, Clarke GH, Nicolaides AN. Quantification of venous reflux by means of duplex scanning. J Vasc Surg 1989; 10: 670–7.
- Vasdekis SN, Clarke HG, Nicolaides AN. Quantification of venous reflux using duplex scanning. In: Davy A, Stemmer R, eds. Proceedings of the Xth World Meeting of the Union Internationale de Phlébologie, London, 1989. Montrouge: John Libbey Eurotext, 1989: 344.
- Weiss, RA, Weiss MA. Resolution of pain associated with varicose and telangiectatic leg veins after compression sclerotherapy. J Dermatol Surg Oncol 1990; 16: 333–6.

Patients with any form of venous disease, from telangiectatic veins to venous ulceration, may benefit from conservative measures designed to decrease venous distension and reduce ambulatory venous hypertension. The severity and type of the medical problem will indicate which of these interventions should be prescribed. A patient handout, such as that shown at he end of this chapter, may be helpful, and repeated encouragement and discussion of these measures by the physician or staff member may increase patient compliance. All of the following interventions have been found to be of potential benefit and are based on pathophysiologic principles and actual patient experience.

Exercise of the lower extremities, particularly weight-bearing activities that emphasize ankle flexion, activates the musculovenous pump and causes the blood to be expelled from the leg veins toward the heart. This provides a period of time during which the pressure within the venous system is lowered and strengthens the muscles so that they become more efficient in pumping the blood out of the legs. Ideally, at least a 30-minute period of continuous exercise should be performed daily. Many patients, however, will be resistant to this change in their level of activity and will cite many reasons why they are unable to comply with this prescription. For these patients, as well as those patients who are truly deconditioned, it is advisable to suggest a modest beginning regimen, such as 5 minutes per day. This can be increased gradually as their exercise tolerance and/or enjoyment of the regimen increases. Most patients will notice a significant reduction in symptoms within several weeks of beginning or increasing an exercise program.

Since many patients spend at least a portion of their day in sitting or standing activities, it is wise for them to consciously activate their musculovenous pump whenever possible. The Basle study[1] demonstrated a clear, exponential rise in the prevalence of venous disease as the amount of daily movement was reduced. Thus, we might be able to reduce the expression of this disease if we mimic the increased venous flow and

reduced pressure that occurs during a day of constant walking by having the patient flex their ankles repetitively during the day. The patient should flex the ankles 5–10 times every few minutes, and walk for 1–2 minutes every 30 minutes throughout the day in order to avoid the prolonged venous congestion that occurs when the feet are dependent and at rest for hours at a time.

Because the full contraction of the muscles involved in pumping the venous blood to the heart requires ankle flexion, the wearing of high heels may reduce venous emptying and cause leg aching or tiredness. Patients should be advised to avoid high heels whenever possible. Some of them will notice a marked improvement in how their legs feel even with this simple intervention.

Raising the feet above the level of the heart for 15–30 minutes several times per day may reduce symptoms and edema. Unfortunately, this intervention is impractical for most people. This may be an effective aid for pregnant women, especially those suffering from symptomatic vulvar varicose veins. It might also be prescribed once daily for those patients who experience pain in their legs after a full day at work, before they proceed with other activities in the home. If patients have significant edema, they might benefit from placing 2- to 3-inch blocks under the legs at the foot of their bed, in an attempt to provide a mild Trendelenburg position through the night. Contraindications to this position include congestive heart failure, gastro-esophageal reflux, chronic obstructive pulmonary disease, sleep apnea, etc.

Compression has many benefits in patients with venous disease.[2-6] It reduces the diameter of the veins, thereby increasing flow velocity and decreasing the chance of thrombosis. It also activates the fibrinolytic activity in the blood, with the same result. It reduces filtration of fluid out of the intravascular space and improves lymphatic flow, thus reducing edema. Graduated compression reduces reflux and improves venous outflow, thus decreasing venous pressure at rest and with ambulation. Compression is also anti-inflammatory, yielding improvement in pain and swelling. Some of these effects last for a period of time after the compression is removed. There are three main types of compression: elastic compression stockings or bandages, inelastic compression garments or bandages, and pneumatic compression pumps. Each has its place in the treatment of venous disease and may be complementary in a given patient.

To properly prescribe compression therapy, it is important to understand the effect of elastic and inelastic compression on venous flow. Venous emptying has two phases: the first is the working phase, during which the muscles contract and the blood is forced through the venous valves, up through the deep veins, toward the heart. During the next phase, the resting phase, the muscles relax and the pressure in the deep veins decreases, allowing blood to move from the superficial veins, through the perforating veins into the deep veins.

In the face of elastic compression, as the muscles swell during their contraction, they expand the stocking. During the resting phase, when the pressure within the deep venous system needs to be low in order to facilitate the movement of blood from the superficial venous system, the elastic recoil of the stocking results in an increase in this venous pressure, thus reducing the filling of the deep veins. In this way, the efficiency of the musculovenous pump is reduced in some patients by the use of elastic compression stockings.

In contrast, inelastic compression augments the emptying of the veins by providing a rigid envelope around the leg. This allows all of the force of the muscular contraction to be directed inward, emptying the deep veins. During the resting phase, the inelastic compression garment offers no compression to interfere with the necessary influx of blood into the deep venous system.

Although inelastic compression is, scientifically, a better form of compression, in practice it is more difficult to apply and maintain. One may use a short stretch bandage (not an ACE® bandage, which has a great deal of elastic in it) and teach the patient or a family member to apply it properly. Ideally, the leg should be elevated when the bandage is placed. The bandage should be applied by simply wrapping the leg, without a lot of tension. If the patient has a lot of edema when the bandage is placed, it will need to be reapplied several times each day, as the edema resolves.

The CircAid® (CircAid Medical Products, Inc., San Diego, CA) is composed of a series of nylon strips that circle the leg and are fastened together with Velcro, allowing the patient to easily adjust the tension on their leg (Figure X). It is available in ready-fit or custom sizes and may be ordered for the calf only, including the thigh, or including a boot for the foot. It is quite durable and is guaranteed for 1 year, making its cost quite reasonable. In theory, inelastic compression is more helpful than elastic compression in patients with serious forms of venous disease such as venous ulceration, chronic venous insufficiency, and intractable symptoms due to varicose veins.

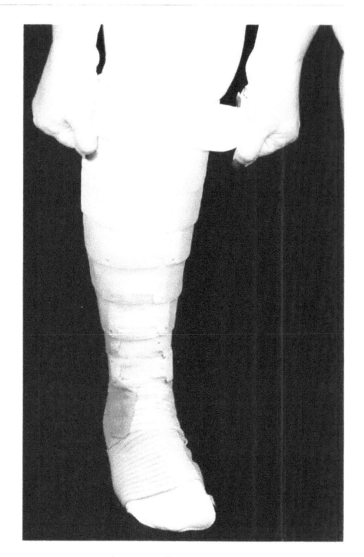

CircAid® Ready-Fit™ Classic-Flex™, the CircAid® system utilizes a series of nylon strips to achieve an inelastic compressive device around the leg. (Image courtesy and copyright of CircAid Medical Products, Inc., San Diego, CA)

In practice, however, elastic compression is used much more commonly. This is because it is generally easy to apply and in fact helps most patients. In addition, since stockings are now more comfortable and available in aesthetically acceptable forms, compliance is better than with inelastic compression garments. For patients with symptoms such as aching or pain due to telangiectatic veins, varicose veins, or chronic venous insufficiency, elastic compression stockings may reduce the severity of their symptoms and retard the progression of their disease. Elastic compression stockings come in four classes, based on the pressure generated by the stocking at the ankle level (Table X), and are graduated (Figure X).

Stockings that are poorly fitted may actually generate a reverse gradient, leading to a "tourniquet effect" that may produce the opposite effect on blood flow. Thus, patients should be measured and fitted according to the charts created by each stocking company. Patients whose measurements fall outside of the ranges on these charts should be fitted with a custom-

Classes of elastic compression stockings

Class	Pressure (approximate)	Suggested indications
I	20–30 mmHg	Aching, swelling, telangiectasias, reticulars
II	30–40 mmHg	Symptomatic varicose veins, chronic venous insufficiency (CVI), post-ulcer
III	40–50 mmHg	CVI, post-ulcer, lymphedema
IV	50–60 mmHg	CVI, post-ulcer, lymphedema

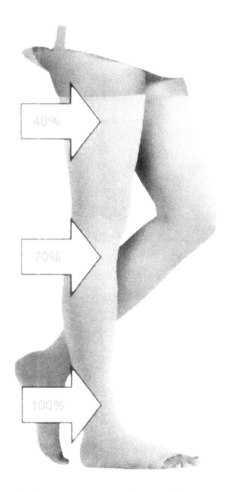

Elastic compression stockings: 100% of the stated pressure should be generated at the ankle level, 70% should reach at the upper calf, and 40% at the thigh level. This creates a gradient which enhances venous reflux and facilitates venous out flow.

RECOMMENDATIONS FOR BETTER LEGS

REGULAR EXERCISE

Walking, running, Stairmaster, aerobics, swimming, elliptical machine, or biking for 30 minutes, 5–7 days per week will help reduce aching, pain, and tiredness in your legs.

ELEVATE YOUR LEGS

Elevating your legs above heart level for at least 10 minutes once or twice daily may diminish aching and swelling.

MOVE YOUR LEGS FREQUENTLY

Flexing your ankles 10 times will pump the blood out of your legs like walking does. Repeat this every 10 minutes while standing or sitting and try to walk for at least 2 minutes every half-hour.

AVOID WEARING HIGH HEELS

Wearing high heels interferes with the normal pumping action that occurs when you walk and may lead to aching and cramping of the legs.

MAINTAIN A PROPER WEIGHT

Even moderate weight loss may reduce aching in the legs due to varicose veins and diminish the rate at which spider veins develop.

WEAR SUPPORT HOSE

Available at pharmacies and medical supply stores. There are many brands to choose from. Lighter support stockings are available at department stores. However, it is best to wear a stocking that is labeled "graduated" as this will really help to improve your vein function.

Light support: 4–14 mm
Heavy support: 20–30 mm
Moderate support: 15–20 mm
Prescription strength: 30–40 mm or above

References

1. Widmer LK. Peripheral venous disorders: prevalence and socio-medical importance. Observations in 4529 apparently healthy persons. Basel Study III. Bern: Hans Huber, 1978; 43–50.
2. Goldman MP, Bergan JJ, Guex JJ. Compression hosiery, compression bandages, and pressure pads. In: Sclerotherapy: Treatment of Varicose and Telangiectatic Leg Veins, 4th edn. St Louis, MO: Mosby, 2007. Appendix A.
3. Christopoulos DG, Nicolaides AN, Szendro G, et al. Air-plethysmography and the effect of elastic compression on venous hemodynamics of the leg. J Vasc Surg 1987; 5: 148–59.
4. Pierson S, Pierson D, Swallow R, Johnson G Jr. Efficacy of graded elastic compression in the lower leg. JAMA 1983; 249: 242–3.
5. Horner J, Fernandez J, Fernandes E, Nicolaides AN. Value of graduated compression stockings in deep venous insufficiency. BMJ 1980; 280: 820–1.
6. Prandoni P, Lensing AW, Prins MH et al. Below knee elastic compression stockings to prevent the post-thrombotic syndrome: a randomized, controlled trial. Ann Intern Med 2004; 141: 249–56.

There are several important principles in the evaluation and treatment of patients with venous disease. The widespread adoption of these concepts has led to a more comprehensive, methodical approach to these patients, and this has subsequently resulted in significant improvements in the quality of care.

Patients with venous disease should be evaluated as any medical patient – with a history of the problem, past medical history, listing of current and prior medications, family history, and review of systems. The physical examination should be performed in a standing position and should include the entire leg(s) from groin to ankle, as well as an examination to the umbilicus if indicated. Doppler and duplex ultrasound examinations should also be performed in the standing position.

Once the extent of the patient's venous disease has been diagnosed, a treatment plan may be formulated. All patients should be given information regarding conservative therapy, to include exercise, weight optimization, and compression, as a minimum.

Patients with venous ulceration require duplex ultrasound examination. The mainstay of treatment for all patients with ulcers is compression. Treatable abnormalities within the superficial venous system should be corrected, if possible. Lifelong compression should be encouraged in all patients who have had venous ulcers.

In general, veins are treated in the following order:

1. Saphenous vein trunks
2. Saphenous vein tributaries
3. Varicose veins unconnected to insufficient saphenous veins
4. Reticular veins
5. Telangiectatic veins

Treatment modalities that have been found to be effective for the various segments of the superficial venous system include the following:

Saphenous vein trunks

1. Thermal ablation: radiofrequency or laser
2. Chemical ablation (ultrasound-guided sclerotherapy)
3. Ligation and stripping

Saphenous vein tributaries

1. Ambulatory phlebectomy

2. Thermal ablation
3. Chemical ablation (ultrasound-guided)
4. Trivex
5. Sclerotherapy

Varicose veins unconnected to saphenous vein trunks

1. Ambulatory phlebectomy
2. Chemical ablation (ultrasound-guided sclerotherapy)
3. Sclerotherapy
4. Trivex

Reticular veins

1. Sclerotherapy
2. Ambulatory phlebectomy

Telangiectatic veins

1. Sclerotherapy
2. Laser

It is important for both the practitioner and the patient to keep in mind that superficial venous disease is an inherited disorder that is chronic and progressive. Any treatment method is at best palliative, as the patient will generally develop insufficiency in other veins as time passes. All of the above treatments have a certain degree of failure, but this may be minimized if the principles of performing a proper and thorough evaluation prior to treatment planning and of treating reflux beginning with the proximal sources before those more distal are followed. Education of patients regarding the importance of minimizing sedentary behaviors, weight control, regular exercise, and the use of graduated compression will also help to diminish the frequency and severity of recurrence.

It is wise to inform patients with significant deep or superficial vein reflux of the potential for venous ulceration and to instruct them in the pre-ulcerative skin changes associated with chronic venous insufficiency so they may present for treatment prior to the development of an ulcer.

For women of childbearing age, it is often advisable to intervene and correct the superficial incompetence prior to the next pregnancy, rather than waiting until childbearing is complete as recommended in the past. This new approach reflects the relative ease of providing more effective treatments than previously.

Goals of sclerotherapy

When we treat varicosities and telangiectasias, we want to remove or obliterate the abnormal vessels that carry retrograde flow, without damaging adjacent or connected vessels that carry normal antegrade flow. Obliterating a vessel is not easy: a small amount of damage will produce intravascular thrombus, but thrombosis alone usually does not result in obliteration of the vessel. Intact endothelium aggressively lyses thrombus, and a thrombosed vessel with intact endothelium will not be sclerosed. See Figure 3.1

Recanalization of thrombosed vessels

Vascular fibrosis and obliteration only occur in response to irreversible endothelial cellular destruction and exposure of the underlying subendothelial cell layer. If an injected sclerosant is too weak, there may be no endothelial injury at all. If the sclerosant is a little stronger, the vessel is damaged, but recanalization occurs and an incompetent pathway for retro-

grade blood flow persists. If the injected sclerosant is too strong, the varicose vessel endothelium is destroyed, but the sclerosant also flows into adjacent normal vessels and causes damage there as well. The key goal is to deliver a *minimum* volume and concentration of sclerosant that will cause irreversible damage to the endothelium of the abnormal vessel, while leaving adjacent normal vessels untouched. It is important to protect normal superficial vessels, and it is critically important to avoid injuring the endothelium of deep veins, because deep vein thrombosis (DVT) places patients at risk of death from thromboembolism, as well as causing permanent disability from chronic deep venous valvular insufficiency. The successful treatment of varicosities and telangiectasias by chemical sclerosis depends upon our ability to produce vascular endothelial damage that is irreversible in the area under treatment, but that does not extend to adjacent normal vessels.

To limit endothelial injury to a controlled area, we exploit differences in flow dynamics between the abnormal veins being injected with sclerosant and the adjacent normal vessels that should not be sclerosed. A thorough understanding of the mechanism of action of the sclerosing agent is essential, as is

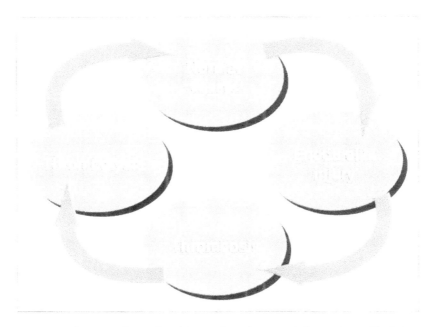

Process of endothelial injury, thrombosis, and thrombolysis. Illustration courtesy of Craig F. Feied

23

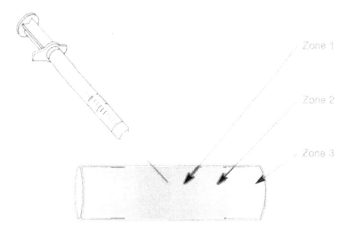

Zone 1

Zone 2

Zone 3

Zones of action of injected sclerosant. (Illustration courtesy of Craig F Feied *et al*)

a firm grasp of the biophysical principles underlying the techniques of sclerotherapy.

Volume dilution and patient positioning

Sclerosant is diluted with blood as it diffuses away from the site of injection, thus if a strong sclerosant is injected there will be three zones of action (Figure 5.2). In zone 1, vascular endothelium is irreversibly injured: the vessel will be fully sclerosed and eventually will be completely replaced by a fibrous tissue. In zone 2, vascular endothelium is injured, and the vessel will be partially or completely thrombosed but will eventually recanalize. In zone 3, the sclerosant will be diluted below its injurious concentration, and there will be no endothelial injury.

Dilution by diffusion from injection site

Because dilution of the sclerosant with blood occurs immediately upon injection, the original injected concentration of sclerosant is not as important as the diluted concentration at the surface of the endothelium. An injected concentration that is perfectly effective in a spider vein (where sclerosant displaces blood rather than mixing with it) may be ineffective in a reticular feeding vein or a truncal varix simply because dilution reduces the final concentration so low that there will be no endothelial injury whatsoever (no zone 1 or 2). If the injected concentration is too high, dilution will leave the final concentration so high that endothelial damage will occur where it is not wanted (zones 1 and 2 are too large). If the injected concentration is just right, dilution will leave a final concentration that is sufficient to injure the local varicose endothelium, but not high enough to damage normal superficial or deep veins (most of the varicose vessel falls into zone 1, a small amount falls into zone 2, and all normal vessels fall into zone 3).

When we select a particular volume and concentration of a chemical agent with which to sclerose a vessel, we are explicitly or implicitly adjusting the injected concentration and volume to take into account the dilution that will occur when the sclerosant is mixed with blood immediately after injection. We also must take into account the further dilution that will occur as the sclerosant flows or diffuses away from the site of injection. The importance of patient positioning in determining dilutional volume often is not properly appreciated by the novice in phlebology.

Because of the cylindrical geometry of blood vessels, the volume contained in a vessel depends on the square of the vessel radius, the volume of any cylinder is calculated as $\pi r^2 L$ (where r is the radius and L is the length of the vessel). Vessels collapse to a smaller radius when the legs are elevated; thus, the volume contained is reduced dramatically. For this reason, the position of the patient has a very powerful effect on the final diluted concentration of sclerosant at the surface of the vessel endothelium (Figure 5.2).

Effect of position on varicose geometry (Figure 5.4)

Standing

For a standing patient with a superficial varicosity 2 cm in diameter, the final concentration at a distance from the injection site of 10 cm (4 inches) is 30 times lower than the initial concentration. Doubling the initial concentration serves only to double the final concentration, which will still be 15 times weaker than the concentration in the syringe. In other words, if 1 cm³ of a 3% solution is injected, the final concentration at the endothelial surface is 1% at a distance of 1 cm from the injection point, 0.5% at a distance of 2 cm, 0.25% at a distance of 4 cm, and 0.2% at a distance of 5 cm (2 inches) from the injection point. As we shall see, this means that it is very difficult to achieve sclerosis of a large vessel by injecting detergent sclerosants with the patient in a standing position: if the highest available concentration is injected, the dilution factor

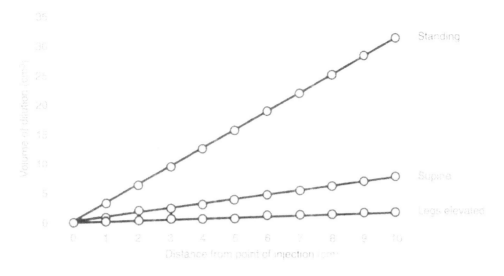

Effect of position on volume of dilution. Illustration courtesy of Craig F. Feied

may still drop the final concentration below the threshold of effectiveness within 1.5 inches from the injection site.

Supine

What about the supine position? Varicose veins that bulge when the patient is standing may collapse when the patient is supine, but duplex ultrasound readily demonstrates that the veins are not empty of blood. Both varicose and normal veins contain a significant volume of blood with the legs extended in the supine position. A bulging varicosity that has a diameter of 2 cm in the standing position may have a diameter of 1 cm in the supine position and of 0.5 cm or less when the legs are elevated as high as possible. With such a patient in the supine position, injection of 1 cm³ of a 1% solution leads to a final concentration of approximately 0.5% at a distance of 1 cm and a concentration of about 0.1% at a distance of 5 cm (2 inches). This supine technique limits dilution enough to allow successful sclerosis of large vessels with detergent solutions, so long as sufficient concentrations and volumes of sclerosants are injected. The only problem is that if an injection of sclerosant at a high initial concentration is made directly into a perforating vessel, so that sclerosant flows directly into the deep system, dilution within the deep vessel will still permit zone 1 and 2 endothelial injury for a short distance within the deep vein. This can lead to deep venous damage and chronic venous insufficiency, to DVT, and to life-threatening pulmonary embolism.

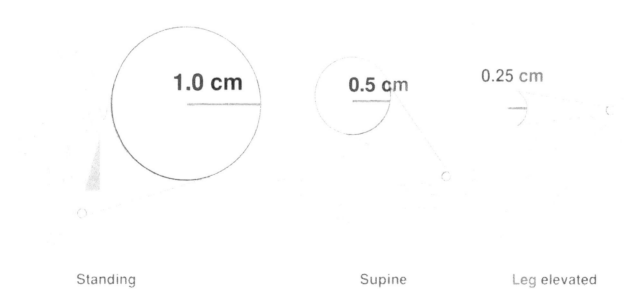

| Standing | Supine | Leg elevated |

Effect of position on vessel size. Illustration courtesy of Craig F. Feied

Legs elevated

In contrast to the standing and supine positions, when a patient lies supine and the legs are raised vertically so that they are well above the central circulation, most superficial varices collapse to the point where they no longer contain any significant volume of blood. Repeating the calculation above for a patient in this position, injection of 1 cm³ of a 3% solution leads to a final concentration of 2.5% at a distance of 1 cm from the injection, and a final concentration of 1.6% at a distance of 5 cm (2 inches). In fact, the final concentration will still be above 1% at a distance of 10 cm from the injection site. Because the superficial varicosity is collapsed, there is very little dilution with distance so long as the sclerosant stays within the floppy-walled varicosity.

With the increasing use of foamed preparations of sclerosants, another factor must be taken into consideration, since the dilution of these medications is significantly reduced. While all of the above considerations still play an important role, the distance over which a foamed sclerosant remains at high concentration is markedly increased. Therefore, smaller volumes and/or lower original concentrations should be employed when using a foamed sclerosant.

What happens when sclerosant passes through into normal vessels? Although flow measurements reveal little or no spontaneous flow through varices and smaller superficial veins when the patient is in the leg-up position, a substantial intravenous volume and a substantial rate of flow still persists in the deep veins and in normal larger superficial veins, which have less collapsible walls. This difference in volumes and flow rates may be exploited to cause damage that is almost perfectly localized to superficial varices. If an elevated, empty varicose vessel is perfused with a concentration of sclerosant so low that it is just barely sufficient to cause endothelial injury, then any further dilution will reduce the concentration below the threshold of injury. Because larger superficial vessels and deep vessels continue to carry a volume of blood in the leg-up position, any sclerosant passing into these vessels will immediately be diluted to a safe and noninjurious concentration, sparing the endothelium of vessels that we wish to preserve. Injection of this "threshold" concentration directly into a perforating vein (or even directly into a deep vein) will not cause any deep vein injury.

Types of sclerosants

Virtually any foreign substance can be utilized to cause venous endothelial damage. Historical methods for producing venous endothelial trauma have included "a slender rod of iron," reportedly used by Hippocrates himself, absolute alcohol, introduced by Monteggio and by Leroy D'Etoilles in the 1840's, and ferric chloride, introduced by Charles-Gabriel Pravaz in 1851. Early sclerosing agents caused many deaths from sepsis and from pulmonary embolism, as well as a high incidence of allergic reactions, local tissue necrosis, pain, and failed sclerosis.

The perfect sclerosant

The best imaginable sclerosant would have no systemic toxicity. It would be effective only above some threshold concentration, so that its effects could be precisely localized through dilution. It would require a long period of contact to be effective, so that it would be relatively more effective in areas of stasis and relatively safer in the deep veins where there is high flow. It would be non-allergenic. It would be strong enough to sclerose even the largest vessels, yet it would produce no local tissue injury if extravasated. It would not cause staining or scarring. It would not cause telangiectatic matting. It would be perfectly soluble in normal saline. It would be painless upon injection. It would be inexpensive. It would be approved by the United States Food and Drug Administration (FDA).

No currently available sclerosant possesses all of the attributes of the perfect sclerosing agent. All currently available sclerosants fall short in one way or another, yet the variety of available agents is such that virtually every situation in which sclerotherapy is indicated can be safely and effectively handled by one or another of the available sclerosants, used alone or in combination.

Detergents

In the 1930's, the class of drugs known as detergents, or as fatty acids and fatty alcohols, came into use with the introduction of sodium morrhuate and sodium tetradecyl sulfate. Detergent sclerosants work by a mechanism known as protein theft denaturation, in which an aggregation of detergent molecules forms a lipid bilayer in the form of a sheet, a cylinder, or a micelle, which then disrupts the cell surface membrane and may steal away essential proteins from the cell membrane surface.

The loss of these essential cell surface proteins causes a delayed cell death; when endothelial cell membranes are exposed to detergent micelles, irreversible cellular morphological changes are seen within minutes by scanning electron microscopy, but the fatal cellular changes that are visible by normal light microscopy do not become apparent for many hours. Unlike many other agents, the detergent sclerosants do not cause hemolysis, nor do they provoke direct intravascular coagulation.

Determinants of activity of detergent solutions

Concentration

At low concentrations, most detergent molecules are individually dissolved in solution, and there are very few micellar aggregates. When the concentration reaches some threshold (known as the critical micellar concentration, CMC) nearly all further detergent molecules added to the solution will enter into micelles. Micelles can cause protein theft denaturation, but individual detergent molecules have no toxicity to the vascular endothelium; thus, for each detergent sclerosant, there is some threshold concentration below which the agent causes no injury. This physical property means that detergent sclerosants offer significant benefits over most of the agents previously used, because they are potent agents that nonetheless have a clear-cut threshold below which they have absolutely no injurious effect on venous endothelium.

Temperature

The solubility of detergents is inversely temperature-dependent. Detergent molecules are much more soluble in cold solutions than in hot ones. This effect is easily seen in everyday life: dishwashing detergent produces a large amount of persistent foam in warm water, while cold water rinses away the soapy foam easily. The solubility of sclerosing agents such as polidocanol is likewise much higher in cold solutions, and because single dissolved molecules are ineffective, the strength of the sclerosing effect is higher at warmer temperatures.

Mixing

Detergent micellar formation can reach a maximum level based upon the temperature and upon the concentration of the detergent in solution. Micellar formation is a steric process, however, and the geometry of macroassemblages often prevents maximal micellar formation. The surface area of lipid bilayer structures such as sheets, cylinders, and micelles is maximized when the solution is shaken to produce a foam. Because it is the surface of these structures that causes protein theft denaturation, a solution that has been shaken will be a more effective sclerosant than one that has not. Unfortunately, foamy bubbles that are injected into spider veins or varicose veins can pass through a patent foramen ovale to lodge in the ocular and cerebral circulation, where they have produced temporary ischemic attacks with temporary blindness and other central nervous system effects.

Currently available detergent agents

Sodium morrhuate

This detergent sclerosant is made up of a mixture of saturated and unsaturated fatty acids extracted from cod liver oil. It was introduced in 1920's, and is still available today. Because it was in general use before there was any requirement to demonstrate safety or efficacy it has been exempted from the need for approval by the FDA for sale in the United States, but there are several problems with the product that make it a less than ideal agent for sclerotherapy. It is a biological extract rather than a synthetic preparation, and the composition varies somewhat from lot to lot. Its components have been incompletely characterized, and a significant fraction of its fatty acids and alcohols are of chain lengths that probably do not contribute to its effectiveness as a sclerosant. It is unstable in solution, causes extensive cutaneous necrosis if extravasated, and has been responsible for many cases of anaphylaxis.

Ethanolamine oleate

Ethanolamine oleate, a synthetic preparation of oleic acid and ethanolamine, has weak detergent properties because its attenuated hydrophobic chain lengths make it excessively soluble and decrease its ability to denature cell surface proteins. High concentrations of the drug are necessary for effective sclerosis, and its effectiveness in esophageal varices depends upon mural necrosis. Allergic reactions are uncommon, but there have been reports of pneumonitis, pleural effusions, and other pulmonary symptoms following the injection of ethanolamine oleate into esophageal varices. Like sodium morrhuate, this agent was exempted from the need for approval by the FDA for sale in the United States. The principal disadvantages of the drug are a high viscosity that makes injection difficult, a tendency to cause red cell hemolysis and hemoglobinuria, the occasional production of renal failure at high doses, the possibility of pulmonary complications, and a relative lack of strength compared with other available sclerosants.

Sodium tetradecyl sulfate

Sodium tetradecyl sulfate (sodium 1-isobutyl-4-ethyloctyl sulfate) is a synthetic long-chain fatty acid salt that has seen extensive industrial use as a synthetic surfactant (soap). It is sold for medical use as a solution of up to 3% concentration with 2% benzoyl alcohol used as a stabilizer. It is effective as a venous sclerosing agent in concentrations from 0.1% to 3%. Like sodium morrhuate and ethanolamine oleate, it was "grandfathered" by the FDA for sale in the United States, but its approval was rescinded at the request of the manufacturer, not for reasons of product safety. In the United States, it is currently available only through compounding pharmacies. Unlike sodium morrhuate, sodium tetradecyl sulfate has proven to be a reliable, safe and effective sclerosant. The principal clinical problems with the drug are a tendency to cause hyperpigmentation in up to 30% of patients, a significant incidence of epidermal necrosis upon extravasation of higher concentrations, and occasional cases of anaphylaxis.

Polidocanol

Polidocanol (hydroxypolyethoxydodecane) is a synthetic long-chain fatty alcohol. All commercially available formulations contain some small quantity of ethanol. The drug was originally developed and marketed in the 1950's under the name Sch 600 as a non-amide, non-ester local anesthetic, was first used as a sclerosing agent in Germany in the 1960's, and was quickly adopted for that use in most countries. The drug was never approved by the FDA for sale in the United States as a sclerosing agent. It is available from local compounding pharmacies. Polidocanol is painless upon injection, does not produce necrosis if injected intradermally, and has been reported to have a very low incidence of allergic reactions. The drug has been intensely studied and extremely well characterized, and has a high therapeutic index. The LD50 in rabbits is 200 mg/kg (approximately 5 times greater than that of procaine), and the LD50 in mice is even greater, at 1200 mg/kg. For human use, the German manufacturer of polidocanol recommends a maximum daily dose of 2 mg/kg, although at least one author has reported the routine use of much higher doses. For all its advantages, polidocanol is not without problems as a sclerosant. Occasional anaphylactic reactions have been reported. In some patients, it may produce hyperpigmentation, although to a lesser extent than many other agents. Telangiectatic matting after sclerotherapy with polidocanol is as common as with any other agent.

Glycerin

Glycerin (glycerol) is a polyalcohol that often is considered a chemical irritant sclerosant. It is classified here with the detergents because it is similar to them in the way in which it causes cell surface protein denaturation. It is very popular in Europe, used as a 72% chromated solution marketed under the name Scleremo. It has not been approved by the FDA, and its use in the United States has only recently become common. Compared with other sclerosants, it is very weak (with approximately one-quarter the strength of polidocanol at the same concentration and volume) and is principally useful in the sclerosis of small vessels. Its principal advantages are that it rarely causes hyperpigmentation or telangiectatic matting and that it very rarely causes extravasation necrosis. The main problems with glycerin are that it is hard to work with because it is extremely viscous, that it can be quite painful on injection, that the chromate moiety is highly allergenic, and that it has occasionally been reported to cause ureteral colic and hematuria.

Foam sclerosants

With the exception of glycerin, detergent sclerosants can be injected in liquid or foamed preparations. Enhancing the activity of a sclerosant by minimizing the hemodilutional effect is actually not a new modification. With the air-block technique, a small amount of air was injected in the syringe before the sclerosant, displacing the blood and allowing more direct endothelial contact. Foaming of a detergent was reported over 50 years ago, but the technique did not become popular until recently. Foam admixtures have included room air, sterile air, carbon dioxide, and a proprietary mixture presently undergoing investigation. In vitro studies with foam demonstrate an impressive ability to fully occupy tubular structures, circumferentially coating the walls. In vivo utilization monitored by duplex ultrasound imaging reveals a similar circumferential endothelial contact, with early spasm of the injected vein, thus further reducing the volume of dilution and enhancing the distribution of the sclerosant. Multiple studies with various mixtures of air and liquid sclerosant are underway. The results to date have been encouraging.

Strong solutions of hypertonic saline and other salt solutions are part of a class that are often referred to as *osmotic scle-*

rosants. These solutions have long been regarded as causing endothelial death by osmotic cellular dehydration. Although it is true that osmotic dehydration at the point of injection is sufficient to rupture red blood cells and to dehydrate some nearby endothelial cells, the evidence suggests that these sclerosants are effective even after dilution has reduced the osmotic gradient to a level that is far too low to account for the effects seen. Thermodynamic and physical chemical calculations suggest that these and other strong ionic solutions probably work by causing conformational denaturation of cell membrane proteins in situ. Like the detergents, they can be diluted to the point where they have no further cellular toxicity.

Hypertonic and ionic solutions currently in use

Hypertonic saline

Hypertonic saline solutions became popular agents for sclerotherapy after they were adopted for that use by Linser in 1926. The most common preparations are 20% and 23.4% solutions. The principal advantage of the agent is the fact that it is a naturally occurring bodily substance with no molecular toxicity. It has not been approved by the FDA for use in sclerotherapy, but it has been used successfully for that purpose by several generations of physicians. There are several reasons why hypertonic saline is not universally accepted as a desirable sclerosing agent. Because of dilutional effects, it is difficult to achieve adequate sclerosis of large vessels without exceeding a tolerable salt load. It can cause significant pain on injection, and leg cramping after a treatment session. If extravasated, it almost invariably causes significant necrosis. Because it causes immediate red blood cell hemolysis and rapidly disrupts vascular endothelial continuity, hypertonic saline is prone to cause marked hemosiderin staining that is not very cosmetically acceptable. All of these problems can be overcome to some extent by meticulous technique and with experience, but patient satisfaction remains lower than with some other available agents. In an effort to reduce the complications, hypertonic saline has been mixed with procaine and heparin in a compound known as Heparsol. This approach has not proven effective, and is rarely used today.

Sclerodex

Sclerodex is a mixture of 25% dextrose and 10% sodium chloride, with a small quantity of 2-phenylethanol. Primarily a hypertonic agent, its effects are similar to those of pure hypertonic saline, but the reduced salt load offers certain benefits. It is not approved by the FDA for sale in the United States. Like pure hypertonic saline, it is somewhat painful on injection, and epidermal necrosis continues to be the rule whenever extravasation occurs.

Polyiodinated iodine

Polyiodinated iodine (Variglobin, Sclerodine) is a mixture of elemental iodine with sodium iodide, along with a small amount of benzyl alcohol. It is rapidly ionized and rapidly protein-bound when injected, and most likely works by localized ionic disruption of cell surface proteins in situ. In vivo conversion of iodine to iodide renders the solution ineffective as a sclerosant, thus localizing the sclerosing effects to the immediate area of injection. The agent is not approved by the FDA for sale in the United States, but is widely used in Europe. The problems with this agent are its high tendency to cause extravasation necrosis, its limited effectiveness at a distance from the injection site, and the risks of anaphylaxis and of renal toxicity that are associated with ionic iodine solutions.

Other chemical sclerosants exist that probably act by a direct or indirect chemical toxicity to endothelial cells: by poisoning some aspect of cellular activity that is necessary for endothelial cell survival. Such agents are less useful to the extent that they also poison other bodily cells. They also lack another of the key attributes of a good sclerosant: they remain toxic to some degree even after extreme dilution, so that there is no real threshold below which injury will not occur.

Both medical and legal considerations are part of the daily practice of medicine today. The medical aspects have been detailed above and are most important, as each physician must decide on the optimal therapy for any given clinical situation. However, the physician's choice must also take into account both federal and state laws and regulations, as sclerosants that have a long, safe record around the world may not be available in the United States. Sclerosants are available through pharmaceutical companies, which are regulated by the FDA, and through compounding pharmacies, which are regulated by the Pharmacy Boards.

By taking into account FDA approval, state regulations, insurance plans, and malpractice coverage, each physician will be able to make appropriate sclerosant choices. It is wise for the phlebologist to consult all of these bodies for their advice in this matter. States may have laws and regulations in relation to the use of compounding pharmacies. Individual malpractice insurance companies should be contacted to review coverage for various sclerosants, especially if considering off-label use. Medicare has specific regulations regarding billing for drugs that are not approved by the FDA. Finally, the use of any sclerosing agent should begin with an appropriate informed consent to assist the patient in understanding the risks and possible complications. This discussion should include the FDA status of the medications being used, and this discussion should be documented in the chart. Sclerotherapy has proven to be highly effective and safe using a variety of sclerosing agents, and the physician should be well versed in both the medical and legal implications of therapeutic choices.

The guiding principle of modern sclerotherapy is to cause irreversible endothelial injury in the desired location, while avoiding any damage to normal vessels that may be interconnected with the abnormal vessel being treated. The aim is to deliver the minimum volume and minimum concentration of the most appropriate sclerosant, and to inject it under conditions that will achieve the minimum effective exposure. Sclerosant concentration, volume, temperature, mixing, and patient positioning are more important in this endeavor than the choice of the actual sclerosing agent. With attention to these details, an accomplished phlebologist can achieve good results with virtually any currently available sclerosing agent.

Introduction

Treatment of telangiectasias and reticular veins is most commonly requested for cosmetic improvement, although most patients are symptomatic as well and may be surprised at the medical benefit they receive from treatment. Telangiectasias are best defined as flat red vessels between 0.1 mm and 1 mm in diameter. Venulectasias are bluish vessels, sometimes distended above the skin surface, and most often 1–2 mm in diameter. Reticular veins have a cyanotic hue and are usually 2–4 mm in diameter. When a complex of reticular veins and telangiectatic veins is located on the lateral thigh, it is felt to be a vestige of embryonic development and is known as the lateral subdermic plexus of Albanese. Clusters of telangiectatic veins along the medial or lateral ankle regions may be the result of underlying insufficiency of the great (GSV) or small (SSV) saphenous veins, respectively. Clusters of telangiectatic veins along the medial thigh or knee regions may also indicate underlying GSV insufficiency. It may be best to evaluate patients with suspected saphenous vein disease using duplex ultrasound examination prior to sclerotherapy of telangiectatic veins in order to formulate a comprehensive treatment plan.

Pre-sclerotherapy photographic documentation

Photographic documentation is important for both the physician and the patient in order to document the results and efficacy of therapy. Photographs help to assure the patient about the progress of treatment, may be required by the insurance carrier, and are helpful for legal documentation.

Post-sclerotherapy compression/activity considerations

The amount of compression following sclerotherapy of telangiectasias and reticular veins is a controversial issue. However, it is frequently recommended that patients wear a class I (20–30 mmHg) or II (30–40 mmHg) graduated compression stocking for a period of time following treatment. The time prescribed may be 3 days to several weeks. The wearing of compression stockings has been associated with improved results and fewer side-effects such as post-sclerotherapy edema and pigmentation. The utilization of hose that provide 15–20 mmHg compression is a secondary choice in patients who will not tolerate the class I prescription compression.

Walking, riding bicycles, and low-impact aerobics are ideal exercises following sclerotherapy. Patients should perform some lower extremity exercise immediately following treatment and daily thereafter.

Consent

A full consent should be signed prior to beginning treatment. This should include all risks, possible complications, and treatment expectations. It is wise to emphasize that most patients will require multiple treatment sessions and that telangiectatic veins typically recur.

Materials (the sclerotherapy tray)

Materials employed in the treatment of telangiectasias and reticular veins are relatively simple. These include

cotton balls soaked with isopropyl alcohol
protective gloves
3 cm³ disposable syringes
10 cm³ syringes and three-way stopcocks if sclerosant is to be foamed
30–32-gauge disposable transparent hub needles
32-gauge needles or 33-gauge autoclavable disposable angiocaths
cotton balls or beveled compression pads
Transpore and/or hypoallergenic paper tape
clear light source, preferably with a magnifying source
a transilluminator, if desired, to aid in visualization of reticular veins
nitroglycerin paste (for prolonged blanching)
hyaluronidase (for prolonged blanching)
anatomic region diagrammatic flow sheet (flow sheets with segmental numerical division of the legs are helpful in documenting areas that are treated at each treatment session)

There are five basic techniques that may be employed to facilitate the sclerotherapy of telangiectatic and reticular veins.

Aspiration technique

Aspiration of a small amount of blood into the needle hub will ensure that the phlebologist has adequately cannulated the vein. Note that the vein may collapse if aspiration is too strong.

Puncture-feel technique

The "feeling" of perforating the vein wall is another technique modality. This technique is slightly more precarious for beginners; however, it can be mastered with time.

Air bolus technique

Injection of 0.5 cm^3 of air prior to introduction of sclerosant will displace the blood in the vein. Once intravascular access has been confirmed, the sclerosant can be safety injected. Air inadvertently introduced into the tissues is not damaging, as the sclerosant might be. Too strong a push may lead to luminal distention and rupture.

Empty vein technique/patient positioning

The persistence of varicose veins after treatment is usually due to recanalization of the intramural thrombus that develops. Introduction of the sclerosant into an empty vein will reduce the amount of thrombus that can develop. This concept is more important when treating larger veins, but may have a significant impact on the treatment of reticular veins as well. A truly empty vein is not achievable; however, elevating the leg or placing the patient in a mild Trendelenberg position can relatively empty the vein of blood. This technique has the following advantages:

> An empty vein has minimal volume, and therefore the sclerosant undergoes less dilution. Also, a smaller volume of sclerosant is necessary to assure contact with the endothelial surface.
> Lower concentrations of sclerosant can be used, since there is less blood in the vein to dilute the solution.

Use of foamed sclerosant

By foaming a detergent sclerosant, dilution is minimized, and this effectively increases the concentration acting on the endothelium. This will result in a more significant effect. Therefore, foamed sclerosants are rarely used in treating telangiectatic veins and are usually used in treating reticular veins and varicose veins. When using a foamed sclerosant, one should reduce the initial concentration, or side-effects such as excessive inflammation, pigmentation, and matting are more likely to occur.

1. Proximal sites of reflux are treated first.
2. Larger and protruding vessels are treated before smaller veins.
3. An entire varicosity is treated at a given treatment session.
4. Adequate compression should be applied immediately after therapy.
5. Ambulation should begin immediately after treatment.

The concept of utilizing the lowest effective concentration of sclerosant capable of producing effective endosclerosis is important. Typical sclerosant concentrations for treatment of telangiectasias, venulectasias, and reticular veins are given in Table 6.1.

If a poor response occurs, the physician may:

1. Increase the concentration of sclerosant
2. Switch to another sclerosant
3. Re-examine the patient to find a possible source of reflux, previously missed

Injection is carried out utilizing one or more of the previously described techniques. Injection may be carried out with the needle bent at an angle of 15°. Two-hand traction is used by either the sclerotherapist or an assistant to keep the skin taut. Large vessels are injected before smaller vessels, i.e., injection of reticular veins feeding smaller telangiectasias or venules may eradicate these, minimizing side-effects such as pigmentation. Areas of vascular arborization should be treated before single vessels are cannulated. The utilization of alcohol to swab the skin prior to injection will increase the index of refraction and thus make the vessels more visible at the skin surface. Brisk cannulation of veins causes minimal vascular trauma, less vasoconstriction, and less chance of extravasation of blood. A quick introduction of the needle under the skin, followed by another quick puncture of the vein itself, works well. Injection pressure is kept to a minimum by performing the injection slowly in order to prevent vascular distention. A small amount of sclerosant (0.1–0.4 cm^3) should be used at each injection site. Small volumes and low injection pressures will minimize side-effects such as telangiectatic matting, ischemic ulceration, and extravasation. Injections are carried out at approximately 3 cm intervals until the entire vessel has been treated.

It is advisable to have the patient wait for 30 minutes after the first treatment session to assure that there is no evidence of type I immediate hypersensitivity (anaphylaxis). Immediate ambulation during this period may help to reduce the incidence of deep vein thrombosis (DVT).

Suggested sclerosant concentrations for treatment of telangiectasias/reticular veins

Vessel type	Sclerosant	Concentration
Telangiectasias < 1 mm	Hypertonic saline	11.7%
	Sodium tetradecyl sulfate	0.1–0.2%
	Polidocanol	0.25–0.75%
	Glycerin	72.0% mixed 2:1 with 1% lidocaine
Venulectasias 1–2 mm	Sodium tetradecyl sulfate	0.25–0.4%
	Hypertonic saline	15.6–23.4%
	Hypertonic glucose/saline	200 mg/mL dextrose, 100 mg/mL sodium chloride, 100 mg/mL propylene glycol, 8 mg/mL phenoxyalcohol
	Polidocanol	0.5–1%
Reticular veins > 2 mm	Hypertonic saline	15.6–23.4%
	Hypertonic glucose/saline (Sclerodex)	As above
	Sodium tetradecyl sulfate	0.25–0.4%*
	Polidocanol	0.5–1.0%*

*The lower concentration is used if the solution is foamed.

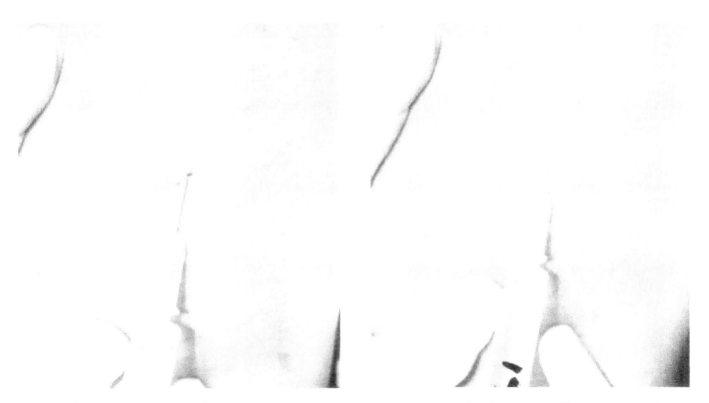

The technique for injection of telangiectasias involves stretching the skin taut, using a 3 cm³ syringe and a 30-gauge needle, and slowly injecting 0.1–0.4 mm³ of the sclerosant as filling of the vessel is observed. (Images courtesy of Helane S Fronek MD)

Spot compression may be applied over injection sites with cotton or gauze pads and micropore tape. Alternatively, beveled foam rubber compression pads may be applied. These compression pads are particularly helpful when treating bulging vessels. Graduated compression, most easily provided through a gradient compression stocking, is suggested in all patients following sclerotherapy and may be all that is necessary to put over the injection sites.

Treatment sessions are carried out at 4- to 12-week intervals to allow enough time to evaluate the results of the prior treatment. It is important to inform patients that most will require several treatments to clear their legs of the unwanted veins. It is also helpful to inform patients prior to beginning their treatment that symptomatic improvement usually occurs quite promptly after successful sclerotherapy, while cosmetic improvement may be more gradual. In patients who have large numbers of telangiectatic veins over much of the surface area of their legs, clearing of their legs may require 1–2 years. It is also important to discuss the likelihood that the patient will develop new telangiectasias with time and that periodic sclerotherapy may be necessary to maintain the desired appearance and/or asymptomatic condition.

Bibliography

Baccaglini H, Spreafico G, Castro C, Sorrentino P. Consensus Conference on Sclerotherapy of Varicose Veins of the Lower Limbs. Phlebology 1997; 12: 2–16.

Badran EL. Techniques for sclerotherapy for sunburst venous blemishes. J Dermatol Surg Oncol 1985; 11: 696–704.

de Groot WP. Practical phlebology — sclerotherapy of large veins. J Dermatol Surg Oncol 1991; 17: 589–95.

Duffy DM. Sclerotherapy. Clin Dermatol 1992; 10: 373–80.

Duffy DM. Small vessel sclerotherapy — an overview. Adv Dermatol 1988; 13: 221–42.

Gallagher PL. Varicose veins — primary treatment with sclerotherapy. J Dermatol Surg Oncol 1992; 18: 39–42.

Goldman MP. Advances in sclerotherapy treatment of varicose and telangiectatic leg veins. Am J Cosmet Surg 1992; 9: 235–40.

Goldman MP. Rational sclerotherapy techniques for leg telangiectasia. J Dermatol Surg Oncol 1993; 12: 933.

Goldman MP, Bennett RG. Treatment of telangiectasia: a review. J Am Acad Dermatol 1987; 17: 167–82.

Goldman MP, Weiss RA, Bergan JJ. Diagnosis and treatment of varicose veins: a review. J Am Acad Dermatol 1994; 31: 393–415.

Guex JJ. Microsclerotherapy. Semin Dermatol 1993; 12: 129–30.

Sadick NS. Sclerotherapy of varicose and telangiectatic leg veins — minimal sclerosant concentration of hypertonic saline and its relationship to vessel diameter. J Dermatol Surg Oncol 1991; 17: 65–70.

Tournay R. How should resistant varicose veins be sclerosed? Phlebology 1990; 5: 151–3.

Weiss MA, Weiss RA. Sclerotherapy. Curr Opin Dermatol 1997; 4: 167–74.

Weiss RA, Goldman MP. Advances in sclerotherapy. Dermatol Clin 1995; 13: 431–45.

Sclerotherapy of varicose veins has been performed since the mid 1800's with varying degrees of success. Advances such as duplex ultrasound pretreatment mapping, intraprocedural ultrasonic guidance, and the foaming of detergent sclerosants have enhanced the predictability of this technique in treating large varicose veins. Sclerotherapy is used commonly as an adjunctive treatment for tributaries of the saphenous vein after endovenous saphenous obliteration by laser or radiofrequency, or after surgical procedures to remove the saphenous trunk. It is also used as primary treatment of nonsaphenous varicosities.

Additionally, by using intraprocedural imaging with ultrasound, sclerotherapy has been used successfully for primary treatment of the saphenous veins themselves. Numerous reports from Europe have demonstrated excellent results with endovenous ablation of the truncal veins using chemical detergent sclerosants, such as polidocanol and sodium tetradecyl sulfate.[1] Successful ablation is reported to be greater than 90%.[2] At least partially because of economic concerns, ultrasound-guided foam sclerotherapy of the truncal and peripheral veins has enjoyed considerable acceptance in Europe and South America. At this time, it remains an investigational, if not intriguing, method of endovenous ablation in the United States. Clinical trials in the United States are planned for the near future.

Many experienced clinicians are comfortable formulating their approach to the patient with venous insufficiency based only on a continuous-wave Doppler examination to provide the "reflux map." However, a thorough duplex ultrasound examination will often provide further insight that may alter one's approach and provide better results. A detailed ultrasound map will afford even greater understanding of the flow and connections of the veins to be treated.

The three classical techniques of sclerotherapy vary in their anatomic targets, and the order in which they are treated:

The Sigg or Swiss method aimed to treat the entire length of the varicose vein.

The Tournay or French method advocated serial injections, beginning with the most proximal site of reflux.

The Fegan approach treated the superficial vein segments overlying incompetent perforator veins only.

Given the current understanding of varicose vein pathophysiology, each technique may find an appropriate application for certain cases.

The aim of modern sclerotherapy is to permanently eliminate all identifiable sources of superficial reflux, starting with the largest refluxing vein.[3] Traditionally, ablation of the superficial veins exhibiting reflux has been a widely accepted prerequisite to achieving this aim. However, experience has shown that sclerotherapy can also provide significant reduction of symptoms when the targeted vein(s) are partially sclerosed and narrowed;[4] this can occur due either to normalization of flow or to attenuation of reflux. Whether surgical or sclerotherapeutic, all treatment of varicose veins is considered palliative, due to the chronicity and natural progression of this disease.[3] Thus, the primary goal is to provide the patient with the longest possible symptom-free interval. Indications for sclerotherapy of varicose veins include leg symptoms due to superficial venous insufficiency; prevention of complications such as hemorrhage, recurrent superficial thrombophlebitis, or leg ulceration; and cosmetic concerns. Contraindications to sclerotherapy may include pregnancy, lactation, allergy to the sclerosing agent, thrombophilia (hypercoagulable state), non-ambulatory status, air travel closely following treatment, and noncompliance.

Injections are accomplished with the patient lying down, with the treated leg either flat or elevated. An appropriate sclerosing agent is used, the concentration of which is determined by the size of the vein to be injected. While polyiodinated iodine and polidocanol are widely used both inside and outside the United States, 0.5–3% sodium tetradecyl sulfate is most commonly used in the United States for treating varicose veins, primarily because it is FDA-approved. Although subacute bacterial endocarditis (SBE) prophylaxis for valvular heart disease and sterile technique are unnecessary precautions, strict OSHA protocol must be followed to protect both patient and sclerotherapist from transmission of bloodborne pathogens. A good practice is to assume that every patient has such infections.

In cases where cannulation is difficult due to the collapse of veins in the supine position, it can be helpful to first outline those veins with a marker while the patient is standing. If cannulation is still difficult with the patient supine, the patient's torso may be elevated, or a tourniquet cuff set at the patient's diastolic pressure can be placed proximal to the area to be treated. Transillumination may also help to define the position of the veins to be treated. Alternatively, cannulation may be performed using small-gauge short-tube butterfly catheters, with the patient sitting or standing. With the needles taped in place, the patient is then placed supine, and injections may be done after intravenous placement by aspiration is reconfirmed.

Smooth and quick cannulation minimizes pain and vessel trauma. If venous blood does not enter the needle hub spontaneously, aspirate first to ensure intravenous placement and then inject slowly over 5–15 s. In general, no more than 1 cm^3 is injected at any site, although 2–3 cm^3 have been used safely when injecting larger veins. Resistance during injection signifies either vasospasm or extraluminal needle placement. Discontinue the injection if repeat aspiration after needle repositioning does not yield free blood flow. Digital pressure proximal and distal to the needle may be used to concentrate the sclerosant within a vein segment. Injections are usually done every 5–15 cm along the treated vein until it exhibits palpable induration and visible contraction. Some phlebologists advocate beginning inferiorly in the leg, with successive injections placed more proximally, in order to take advantage of the normal direction of flow in the vein. This reduces both the amount of sclerosant necessary to treat the veins and the total number of injections, since the sclerosant will travel further along the vein in the antegrade direction than it will when injections are started superiorly in the leg and the sclerosant flows only to the next competent valve. Mild localized erythema as well as induration and swelling of vein segments are commonly observed immediately following the injection. Re-examination immediately after treatment may reveal resistant, unresponsive segments, which can benefit from re-injection.

Three optional enhancement techniques may potentiate the effect of the sclerosant by increasing its contact with the endothelium:

1. The "air block" technique strives to empty the vein by first injecting 0.5 cm^3 of air just prior to injecting the sclerosant.
2. A sclerosant foam can be produced by mixing air or physiologic gas with a detergent sclerosant via a three-way stopcock in a 4:1 ratio.
3. The vein can be massaged immediately after injection to more widely distribute the sclerosant.

A fourth technique thought to act through synergism consists of the sequential injection of two different sclerosing agents into the same vein in one session.

Varicose veins without saphenous reflux

When the saphenous axes are deemed competent, varicose veins are injected directly using the above technique.

Examples of this include isolated saphenous tributary insufficiency (e.g., the anterior circumflex thigh vein) in women, superior external pudendal tributaries, which usually drain from the groin (medial to the saphenofemoral junction) down the buttock and posterior thigh; post-stripping incompetent perforator veins and their tributaries; large posterolateral system venectasias, and vaginal/labial varicosities. Most of these veins respond to 0.4% sodium tetradecyl sulfate, but may require stronger concentrations. It is prudent to use a milder concentration at first, stepping up the concentration only as needed. Nonbulging lateral thigh venectasias 2–4 mm in diameter often respond to lower concentrations of 0.2–0.3% sodium tetradecyl sulfate, with their visible disappearance being used as treatment endpoint. Lower concentrations should be used when a foamed preparation of the detergent sclerosant is being injected.

Varicose veins with saphenous reflux

When visible varicose veins are associated with underlying saphenous reflux, treatment is first directed to the saphenous vein, and then to the surface varicosities. The saphenous veins may be treated surgically or with endovenous ablation procedures, including thermoablation techniques (radiofrequency and laser), and chemical ablation with ultrasound-guided sclerotherapy. Formerly known as ultrasound- or duplex-guided sclerotherapy (UGS or DGS), endovenous chemical ablation has been in use since the 1990's.

As the diagnostic "gold standard" for anatomic and reflux mapping of lower extremity veins, duplex ultrasound also has the potential to improve the safety, accuracy, and efficacy of sclerotherapy of the saphenous veins. UGS utilizes real-time feedback for confirmation of three sequential steps performed under continuous imaging.

1. Intraluminal placement of injecting needle tips or catheter within the targeted, incompetent vein.
2. Intraluminal injection and direct control of the sclerosing agent.
3. Attainment of vasospasm (treatment endpoint).

Such an undertaking is a serious commitment, and should not be taken lightly or without adequate preparation. A tool is only as good as its operator; when used properly, it facilitates the task at hand, but when used casually or without proper training, it may become dangerous and actually multiply the risk due to a false sense of security. Endovenous chemical ablation may be appropriate for any of the following when incompetence is identified, either alone or in combination: great or small saphenous veins; perforator veins; and saphenous tributaries including intersaphenous and Giacomini veins. The limits of this technique remain undefined, and cases of junctional incompetence with saphenous diameters as large as 30 mm have responded. The use of foamed detergent sclerosants has markedly improved the efficacy of this treatment modality over liquid sclerosants. It may be especially helpful for the anatomically variable and complex small saphenous system, post-surgical recurrences, and tributaries that are tortuous and thus not easily cannulated with a catheter. The UGS procedure requires a linear array transducer of appropriate length and frequency to provide high-quality images of the vascular system and surrounding tissues, usually a 7.5–15 MHz transducer. While color flow systems are important in the pretreatment diagnostic evaluation and mapping procedure, grayscale is more commonly used for procedural imaging.[12]

After detailed anatomic mapping with thorough assessment for reflux of both deep and superficial venous systems, the patient lies down with the treated leg positioned for injection. The junction between the vein to be treated and the deep venous system or normal vein can be manually compressed in an attempt to direct the flow of sclerosant into the abnormal vein. When using the standard Tournay technique, 1–3 cm^3 of sclerosant are sequentially injected under ultrasound visualization, starting 3–4 cm distal to the saphenofemoral or saphenopopliteal junction, proceeding distally as previously injected segments are observed to spasm. Alternatively, one may take advantage of the normal flow of venous blood and begin in the distal lower leg, progressing proximally to near the deep vein junction in order to reduce the volume of sclerosant and number of injections. Incompetent perforating veins may be indirectly sclerosed by treatment of their respective overlying superficial vein, and usually do not require direct injection. It is also possible to employ a catheter, placed distally, to deliver a fixed amount of sclerosant to the proximal saphenous vein. When using direct needle injection, it is imperative to maintain continuous visualization of the needle tip in order to determine if, due to movement of the needle or spasm of the vessel, the needle has moved into the vein wall or outside of the vein. If this has occurred, injection is immediately stopped at this site.

Early data on UGS using nonfoamed sclerosant solutions demonstrated an 80% success rate for post-stripping recurrences[5], and a 77–90% success rate at 1–2 years for great and small saphenous incompetence.[5,8–10,13] The more recent introduction of foamed sclerosant preparations has produced additional data substantiating the high success rates anecdotally observed by many practitioners.[1,2,10,11]

Certain factors are thought to affect efficacy and recanalization after sclerotherapy of large varicose veins. Brisk, daily 30- to 60-minute walks are encouraged. Activities that induce Valsalva should be avoided for several weeks, such as lifting heavy weights, resistance training, and vigorous sports requiring forceful straining. Venodilatation from extreme heat, such as saunas and spas, should also be avoided. With hard data lacking, opinions vary widely on the use of such restrictions, which are usually recommended for 1–6 weeks. Because of thrombogenic effects,[14] it is sometimes recommended that long-distance air travel should be avoided immediately following sclerotherapy.

Evacuation of intravascular hematoma helps to relieve pain,

minimize pigmentation, and reduce the chance of recanalization. Depending on the individual patient's response, this is usually done between 2 and 4 weeks post treatment, and again at 6–8 weeks if indicated. Re-accumulation in previously evacuated areas suggests recanalization, as does post-treatment hyperpigmentation associated with pain or telangiectatic matting persisting after 2 months.

The use of compression remains controversial, but is the standard of care at present in the United States. Class II (30–40 mmHg) graduated compression hose is most commonly employed for this purpose, and may be used with or without the addition of a foam pad reinforcement over large, bulging veins. Recent data indicate that a class I (20–30 mmHg) stocking may result in an equivalent benefit. A special situation applies to labial and very proximal thigh varicosities, where standard leg hosiery does not reach. For this purpose, tight-fitting Lycra bicycle shorts with foam pads may be used. The Prenatal Cradle V2 Supporter™ is made expressly for labial varicosities during pregnancy, but works well as a post-treatment compression device.[15]

Regular follow-up is recommended, as varicose vein disease is chronic and progressive, and recurrences as well as new varicosities will inevitably occur. In the management of this diverse disease process, sclerotherapy is an extremely versatile and effective technique that allows the treatment of nearly any abnormal vessel and is well tolerated by most patients.

1. Frullini A, Cavezzi A. Sclerosing foam in the treatment of varicose veins and telangiectases: history and analysis of safety and complications. Dermatol Surg 2002; 28: 11–15.

2. Cavezzi A, Frullini A, Ricci S, Tessari . Treatment of varicose veins by foam sclerotherapy. Phlebology 2002; 17: 13–18.

3. Baccaglini U, Spreafico G, Castoro C, Sorrentino P. Sclerotherapy of varicose veins of the lower limbs. Consensus Paper. North American Society of Phlebology. Dermatol Surg 1996; 22: 883–9.

4. Kuefner G. Normalization of long saphenous flow after ultrasound-guided injections: an acceptable failure. 8th Annual North American Society of Phlebology Congress, Ft Lauderdale, FL, 1995.

5. Kanter A, Thibault PK. Saphenofemoral incompetence treated by ultrasound-guided sclerotherapy. Dermatol Surg 1996; 22: 648–52.

6. Kanter A. Clinical determinants of ultrasound-guided sclerotherapy outcome. Part 1: The effects of age, gender, and vein size. Dermatol Surg 1998; 24: 131–5.

7. Thibault PK, Lewis WA. Recurrent varicose veins. Part 2: Injection of incompetent perforating veins using ultrasound-guidance. J Dermatol Surg 1992; 18: 895–900.

8. Zummo M, Forrestal M. Sclerotherapy of the long saphenous vein – a prospective Duplex controlled comparative study. Phlebology 1995; Suppl 1: 571–3.

9. Marley W. Ultrasound-directed sclerotherapy: 90% closure one year after treating trunkal varices with junctional incompetence. 11th Annual North American Society of Phlebology Congress, Palm Desert, CA, November 1997.

10. Cabrera J, Cabrera J Jr, Garcia-Olmedo MA. Treatment of varicose long saphenous veins with sclerosant in microfoam form: long term outcomes. Phlebology 2000; 15: 19–23.

11. Barrett JM, Allen B, Ockelford A, Goldman MP. Microfoam ultrasound-guided sclerotherapy of varicose veins in 100 legs. Dermatol Surg 2004; 30: 6–12.

12. Thibault Duplex examination. Dermatol Surg 1995; 21: 77–82.

13. Isaacs M, Forrestal M. Sequential ultrasound-guided treatment of trunkal veins. 9th Annual North American Society of Phlebology Congress, San Diego, CA, 1996.

14. Eklof B, Kistner RL, Masuda EM, et al. Venous thromboembolism in association with prolonged air travel. Dermatol Surg 1996; 22: 637–41.

15. Ninia J. Treatment of vulvar varicosities by injection–compression sclerotherapy. Dermatol Surg 1997; 23: 573–5.

Sclerotherapy can be used to treat both small and large varices of the superficial venous system and perforators. Sclerotherapy results can be optimized and the risk of complications minimized by properly selecting the patient, performing accurate physical and ultrasound examinations, and choosing the appropriate sclerosant, sclerosant concentration, sclerosant volume, and injection sites for the vein(s) being treated. Post-treatment instructions, particularly compression and ambulation, are designed to improve the results and safety of sclerotherapy. Adequate understanding of venous anatomy and pathophysiology as well as the ability to prevent, recognize, and treat complications are required before embarking on treatment.

Obviously, treatment should not be done using a sclerosant to which the patient is allergic. Patients at high risk for deep vein thrombosis (DVT) are not good candidates for sclerotherapy. Risk factors to consider include but are not limited to a history of DVT/pulmonary embolism (PE), a family history of venous thromboembolism, hypercoagulable state, long-distance travel, bedrest, and an inability to ambulate. It is best to avoid treatment of patients who are pregnant, who have significant systemic illness, lymphedema, or peripheral arterial insufficiency, or who have unrealistic expectations. Removal of surface varices is contraindicated when they are the only significant outflow tract available in patients with severe deep venous obstruction. This may affect only 10% of those with deep venous obstructive syndromes, as deep venous collaterals are probably more important than superficial collaterals.[1]

Post-treatment instructions are designed to increase efficacy and reduce complications. Patients may be asked to perform dorsiflexions of the ankles before they get off the treatment table. This is to help flush sclerosant that has entered the deep system and to minimize the potential for thrombosis. Compression stockings are then donned. Patients generally wear a class I (20–30 mmHg) or II (30–40 mmHg) stocking, depending on the size of the veins being treated, patient tolerance, and physician preference. Compression needs to be mod-

ified if the patient has significant peripheral arterial insufficiency; in this situation, an inelastic form of compression (short stretch bandages, CircAid, etc.) may be indicated. Stockings are often recommended for 3 days following treatment of small veins and for up to 2 weeks after ultrasound-guided sclerotherapy of saphenous veins. Small studies have demonstrated improved results in patients wearing graduated compression following sclerotherapy, but the results have not been significant. Compression also alleviates the discomfort that may occur following sclerotherapy. It is well known that compression reduces the risk of thromboembolism. Therefore, it is wise from a medical and medicolegal standpoint to recommend compression stockings after sclerotherapy. Note that ACE® bandages are not an adequate form of compression.

Patients are asked to walk for 15–30 minutes before they leave the office area. Walking helps to reduce pressure in the superficial veins as well as increase flow through the deep venous system. This also ensures that patients will be in the office area during the time an allergic reaction would most likely occur. They should continue to exercise a minimum of 30–60 minutes per day, in 15-minute or longer sessions, for 1–2 weeks. Hot baths, Jacuzzis, and lifting heavy weights are also to be avoided.

Sclerotherapy, when performed appropriately, is a remarkably effective and safe technique. However, complications can and do occur. Below is a discussion of the most common as well as the most serious complications.

Post-sclerotherapy hyperpigmentation, due to hemosiderin deposition in the superficial dermis, is the most common adverse effect after sclerotherapy.[2] A brownish discoloration appears, generally within a few weeks after treatment, along the course of the treated vessel in about 10–30% of patients (Figure 8.1). Spontaneous clearing within 6–12 months is typical, although it may occasionally persist for longer than a year.[3]

The claim that certain sclerosants are more likely to cause pigmentation than others is unsubstantiated. However, the incidence of pigmentation is increased if the potency of the sclerosant is too strong for the vein being treated or if proximal reflux is untreated. Patients with high iron stores may be more susceptible to pigmentation.[4] More superficial veins,

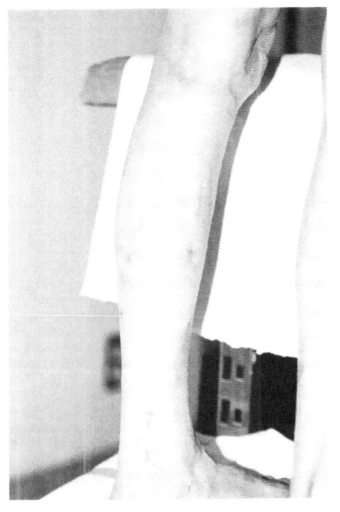

Post-sclerotherapy pigmentation. (Image courtesy of Helane S Fronek MD)

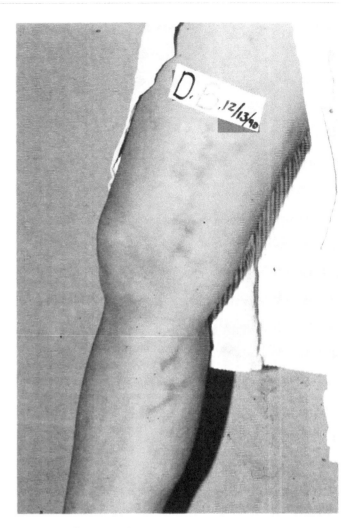

Post-sclerotherapy pigmentation in a patient on minocycline. (Image courtesy of Helane S Fronek MD)

particularly blue veins, pigment more commonly than deeper veins. Small superficial veins (<1 mm in diameter) rarely pigment. Patients on minocycline (Figure 8.2), those with strong, persistent sun exposure, and those taking nonsteroidal anti-inflammatory drugs (NSAIDs) may be at greater risk. Post-sclerotherapy coagula should be drained to reduce the hemosiderin load.

If pigmentation does occur, tincture of time is the treatment of choice. If pigmentation fails to clear within 6–12 months, underlying reflux should be ruled out. Laser treatment may be considered if the pigmentation fails to clear spontaneously. The Q-switched laser may be the most effective laser in this regard. Treatment with chemical peeling agents carries the risk of scarring. Bleaching agents are ineffective, as the pigmentation is not melanocytic.

Swelling

Multiple factors are responsible for swelling after sclerotherapy. Edema is most common when varicose veins or telangiectatic veins below the ankle are treated, especially when volumes greater than 1 cm³ are injected into the ankle or foot and when higher concentrations of sclerosing agents are utilized. It may be caused directly by the application of nongraduated compression following sclerotherapy. Edema may be significantly reduced by the use of graduated compression stockings following sclerotherapy. Edema is usually self-limiting and generally resolves within several days to several months.

Pain

Several variables may be altered to minimize the pain felt by the patient during sclerotherapy. The smallest needle that one is able to use should be utilized, and the needle should be changed frequently. Needles with an acute angle on the bevel and those that are coated with silicone generally result in less pain. The least painful sclerosing agent should be chosen, and diluted with normal (0.9%) saline to the lowest effective concentration. Hypertonic agents frequently cause severe burning and cramping, although this may be lessened with slower injection and by diluting the saline, although the lower concentration will reduce its effectiveness. Injections with sodium tetradecyl sulfate and polidocanol are less painful than injections with osmotic agents. Burning or stinging pain resulting from any sclerosant may be diminished by firm pressure or massage of the affected area.

Topical anesthetic creams may be helpful in small areas, but are usually unnecessary and potentially dangerous when used over a large surface area.

Aching in the legs is common for several hours to days following sclerotherapy, and may be relieved by having the patient walk briskly and by the application of graduated compression stockings immediately following the treatment. Aching that does not respond to these measures may indicate the presence of DVT and should be evaluated.

Telangiectatic matting

"Matting" or "blushing" refers to the appearance of tiny red telangiectasias that appear following vein treatment (Figure 8.3). The incidence of this complication after sclerotherapy is approximately 15%. Spontaneous matting may occur.

The cause of matting remains unclear. It has been suggested that this represents either dilatation of pre-existing subclinical vessels or angiogenesis due to inflammatory processes and vascular obstruction. Partial sclerosis of underlying veins may

also be a contributing factor. Predisposing patient factors may include obesity, a family history of telangiectasias, longer duration of spider veins, and exposure to excess estrogens.

It is widely believed that matting is more common if the sclerosant dosage is too high. Technique-related measures to prevent this complication include using the minimum sclerosant concentration, small volumes, and low pressure when treating a vein.

Although matting may be permanent, it usually resolves spontaneously over several months. The first step in treating matting is to look for untreated proximal reflux from saphenous veins, perforators, tributaries, or reticular veins. Infrared imaging or transillumination may help detect "hidden" reticular veins, while duplex ultrasound can evaluate deeper tributaries, saphenous veins, and perforators. Areas of matting may be treated with "gentle" sclerotherapy using very low injection pressures, injection volumes, and sclerosant concentrations. A variety of lasers/light devices may be used, including the 585 nm pulsed dye laser, the 532 nm long-pulsed laser, intense pulsed light, and the 1064 nm long-pulsed Nd:YAG laser. See Figures 8.4 and 8.5.

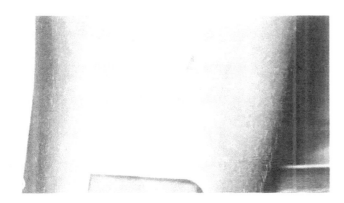

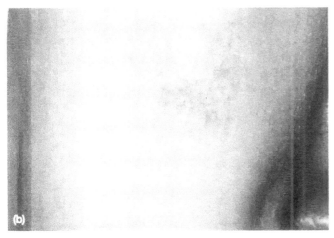

(a) Telangiectasias before sclerotherapy. (b) Telangiectatic matting after sclerotherapy. (Image courtesy of Helane S Fronek MD)

Telangiectatic matting that failed to respond to sclerotherapy and laser treatment. (Image courtesy of Steven E Zimmet MD)

Telangiectatic matting which improved after ultrasound-guided sclerotherapy of an incompetent small saphenous vein. (Image courtesy of Steven E Zimmet MD)

Folliculitis

Occlusion of any hairy area can promote the development of folliculitis, especially if the area becomes moist with perspiration. Treatment consists of removal of the dressing or compression and application of an antibacterial soap or a topical antibiotic gel. The folliculitis usually resolves within a few days. If itching is present, a topical steroid preparation or oral antihistamines may be used. Only rarely will systemic antibiotics be necessary.

Cutaneous necrosis

Cutaneous necrosis (Figure 8.6) is probably the most frequent cause of malpractice actions after sclerotherapy. Although ulceration may occur following the use of any sclerosant, it is more common with hypertonic saline. The cause may be extravasation or injection into an arteriole. One study found that 4% of telangiectasias had a communication with a dermal arteriole. An occluded dermal arteriole was seen on biopsy in a small series of patients with cutaneous ulceration after sclerotherapy.

If extravasation of hypertonic saline or of a large volume of a high concentration of sclerosant occurs, treatment with hyaluronidase (75 units in 3 mL) is advisable. This has been shown in prospective, randomized, and blinded animal studies to significantly reduce the incidence and size of ulceration following intradermal injection of both 23.4% hypertonic saline and 1% sodium tetradecyl sulfate. This protective effect is probably due to enhanced egress of the extravasated solution and an independent ability of hyaluronidase to preserve cellular function. It is not due to dilution.

A porcelain white blanching may develop in the event of arteriolar injury or spasm. There have been anecdotal reports that massage and topical 2% nitroglycerin ointment prevents ulceration.

In addition to the measures discussed above, the risk of ulceration will be minimized with meticulous technique, by using sclerosants other than hypertonic saline, by using minimum sclerosant concentrations and volumes, and by using low injection pressures. In the event of ulceration, the use of an occlusive wound dressing reduces pain and speeds healing. Excision and primary closure can be considered, but are rarely needed and may add to the patient's pain and disfigurement.

Superficial thrombophlebitis

Superficial thrombophlebitis (STP) may occur after sclerotherapy. It occurs primarily after treatment of larger varicose veins, and is heralded by an area of erythema, heat and tenderness over an indurated venous segment. This will usually develop within a few weeks of treatment and may involve the treated area or a venous segment proximal or distal to the injection site. Prophylactic low molecular-weight heparin (LMWH) may be considered when treating patients at significantly increased risk of thromboembolism. The use of appropriate sclerosant concentration and volume as well as post-treatment compression and ambulation may help prevent this complication. Once STP is diagnosed, the possibility of involvement of the proximal saphenous veins and/or concomitant DVT should be considered and ruled out with ultrasound examination if indicated. Compression, ambulation, and NSAIDs generally reduce discomfort and speed resolution. Evacuation of liquefied thrombus is helpful. Bedrest is contraindicated. Prophylactic LMWH should be considered if there is STP of the proximal great saphenous vein. Ligation/division of the saphenofemoral junction should be considered for ascending saphenous thrombophlebitis within 5 cm of the deep system.

Deep vein thrombosis

While DVT has occurred after sclerotherapy, the reported incidence has been less than that seen in the general population. This seems surprising, as sclerotherapy may affect all components of Virchow's triad (endothelial damage, venous stasis, and coagulation). It is likely that this complication is somewhat under-recognized, as DVT may be clinically silent. DVT has even occurred after sclerotherapy of telangiectasias. However, the use of post-sclerotherapy exercise and graduated compression and the higher flow rate in deep veins probably helps to reduce the incidence of DVT. If a DVT develops, the patient should be evaluated for a hypercoagulable state and treatment should be immediately initiated.

Nerve injury

Injury to sensory nerves, such as the saphenous or sural nerve (which lie close to the great and small saphenous veins respectively), may rarely occur following sclerotherapy of deeper venous segments. This may cause temporary or permanent nerve dysfunction. Injury to superficial nerves may also occur

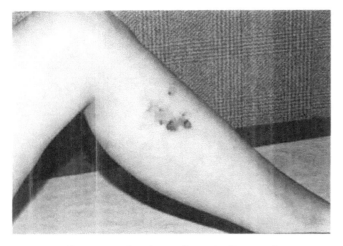

Cutaneous ulcerations after sclerotherapy. (Image courtesy of Helane S Fronek MD)

as a compressive neuropathy due to stockings worn after sclerotherapy. This usually resolves spontaneously. Injury to motor nerves is extremely rare and should be evaluated promptly after it has been diagnosed.

Vasovagal reactions are much more common than anaphylactic reactions and must be differentiated from them. Cardiac arrest has occurred in healthy patients following routine venipuncture.[24] Patients who are vasovagal have bradycardia and diaphoresis, whereas those with anaphylaxis have tachycardia and often pruritus, erythema, hives, and a feeling of doom.

Vasovagal reactions are more common during duplex ultrasound examination with the patient in a standing position than during sclerotherapy. The prodrome typically consists of anxiety, confusion, diaphoresis, nausea, tachypnea, and tachycardia. Bradycardia then develops in the setting of decreased peripheral vascular resistance. Orthostatic hypotension can develop, which may cause loss of consciousness and even clonic seizure activity.

Vasovagal reactions may be prevented by asking the patient to eat prior to treatment, by treating the patient in a supine position, and by allaying the patient's anxiety. If a vasovagal reaction occurs, most patients rapidly improve once placed in a Trendelenburg position. Loss of consciousness should be treated with atropine, up to 1 mg as needed.[25]

Allergic reactions, with an estimated incidence of 0.3%, may occur with any sclerosant.[8] They usually manifest within 30 minutes of treatment, but later onset is possible. These allergic reactions, most of which are immunoglobulin E (IgE)-mediated, may develop with the first treatment, so using a test dose is probably not helpful.

The key to management of allergic reactions is prompt recognition. A protocol to manage these complications should be present in each treatment room. The staff should be knowledgeable about basic resuscitation techniques, and emergency medications and supplemental oxygen should be available. All staff should know how to contact emergency medical services (EMS).

Urticaria may be treated with oral antihistamines. Oral corticosteroids are given if the urticaria do not respond promptly. Any patient with an allergic reaction should be evaluated for wheezing and stridor by auscultating the chest and neck respectively. Vital signs should be assessed and an intravenous (IV) line should be placed in any patient with a potentially serious allergic reaction. Supplemental oxygen should be used as needed. Bronchospasm should be treated with IV antihistamines, corticosteroids, and a bronchodilator. Stridor should also be managed with IV antihistamines and corticosteroids. Intubation may be necessary, and EMS should be activated for

potentially severe reactions. While the patient is still in the office, oxygen should be administered, epinephrine injected (0.3–0.5 cm^3 of a 1:1000 dilution subcutaneously every 10–20 minutes × 3 as required), and 1–2 L of normal (0.9%) saline or lactated Ringer's solution delivered through the IV line. Obviously, patients with serious allergic reactions should be transferred via EMS to a hospital. A more thorough review of anaphylaxis and its management is available.[26, 27]

The most severe reactions may be anaphylactic (IgE-mediated reactions that require previous sensitization) or anaphylactoid (complement- and/or mast cell-mediated that may occur on the first exposure).[28] These two reactions are clinically indistinguishable, and often involve the cutaneous, respiratory, cardiovascular, and gastrointestinal systems. Serum tryptase levels may be obtained and serve as a useful marker for either anaphylactic or anaphylactoid reactions.

Some authors have suggested that allergic reactions to detergent sclerosants, such as sodium tetradecyl sulfate, are often due to solubilization of latex products from the rubber plunger in the syringe in the sclerosant solution.[9] However, there is no evidence that this is the case.

The most feared complications of sclerotherapy are anaphylaxis and intra-arterial injection. Fortunately, these are both rare. Intra-arterial injection can occur even when ultrasound guidance is used. The danger areas for intra-arterial injection include the posterior medial malleolar region, perforators (with their accompanying perforating arteries), and the saphenofemoral and saphenopopliteal junctions, although the arteries at greatest risk in these latter areas are generally not the femoral or popliteal arteries. Instead, the external pudendal artery, a small vessel that can cross anterior to the great saphenous vein, and unnamed superficial arteries near the small saphenous vein are most frequently affected. Arteriovenous anastomoses may explain some cases of arterial injection.[29]

Intra-arterial injection may or may not cause immediate pain.[30] Cutaneous changes, such as erythema, cyanosis, or pallor, typically occur quickly. The consequences of intra-arterial injection range from no sequelae to necrosis of skin, subcutaneous tissue, and/or muscle,[30] rarely leading to amputation. Occlusion of small arteries may lead to the development of a compartment syndrome with resulting nerve damage and even paralysis.

Prevention of this complication requires meticulous technique. When treating veins below the skin using ultrasound-guided techniques, it is important to use high-quality duplex ultrasound machines and to have an appropriate level of expertise in understanding ultrasound images. Once intravenous placement is assured, clear visualization of the needle tip at all times is essential, as the needle may perforate the vein and enter another vessel through operator movement or due to venous spasm. Using catheters or open needles when injecting in a high-risk area may provide more security that the solution is only injected into a vein. Perforators can be treated by injecting the sclerosant into an overlying varicosity and not directly into the perforator. If the patient complains of pain, the injection should be stopped if there is any question or concern.

Intra-arterial injection must be considered a medical emergency. The patient should be hospitalized and consultation obtained with vascular surgery and interventional radiology. Heparin has been shown to prevent postischemic endothelial cell dysfunction, independent of its anticoagulant activity, and has been useful in the treatment of intra-arterial injection of barbiturate. Heparin may also have been helpful in treating intra-arterial injections during sclerotherapy of varicose veins. Fibrinolytic therapy has reportedly been beneficial following the intra-arterial injection of a variety of substances. This may be helpful following intra-arterial injection of a sclerosant, as an obstructive sludge without evidence of spasm or intimal damage has been found after experimental injection of canine arteries with 3% sodium tetradecyl sulfate. Fibrinolytic therapy should be delivered via an intra-arterial line. It has been suggested that antiplatelet agents such as glycoprotein (GP) IIb/IIIa inhibitors may be helpful in reducing the obstructive sludge. Spasm has been noted in at least some cases of intra-arterial injection. It may be reasonable to consider vasodilators in addition to the measures above.

Concluding comments

Sclerotherapy is a remarkably well tolerated and efficacious nonsurgical procedure that can be used to treat both small and large varices of the superficial venous system and perforators. The results of sclerotherapy can be optimized and the risk of complications minimized by obtaining the proper education and training prior to performing the procedure. Patient selection and a wise choice of sclerosant as well as its concentration, volume, and sites for injection are other important considerations. Understanding the potential complications, as well as their prevention, diagnosis, and treatment, is essential. Other publications may be consulted for a more thorough review of these and other complications.

References

1. Labropoulos N, Volteas N, Leon M, et al. The role of venous outflow obstruction in patients with chronic venous dysfunction. Arch Surg 1997; 132: 46–51.

2. Goldman MP, Kaplan RP, Duffy DM. Postsclerotherapy hyperpigmentation: a histologic evaluation. J Dermatol Surg Oncol 1987; 13: 547–50.

3. Georgiev M. Postsclerotherapy hyperpigmentation: a one-year follow-up. J Dermatol Surg Oncol 1990; 16: 608–10.

4. Thibault PK, Wlodarczyk. Correlation of serum ferritin levels and postsclerotherapy pigmentation – a prospective study. J Dermatol Surg Oncol 1994; 20: 684–6.

5. Weiss RA, Weiss MA. Incidence of side effects in the treatment of telangiectasias by compression sclerotherapy: hypertonic saline vs. polidocanol. J Dermatol Surg Oncol 1990; 16: 800–4.

6. Scultetus AH, Villavicencio JL, Kao TC, et al. Microthrombectomy reduces postsclerotherapy pigmentation: multicenter randomized trial. J Vasc Surg 2003; 38: 896–903.

7. Tafazzoli A, Rostan EF, Goldman MP. Q-switched ruby laser treatment for postsclerotherapy hyperpigmentation. Dermatol Surg 2000; 26: 653–6.

8. Ramelet AA, Monti M. Phlebology: The Guide. Amsterdam: Elsevier, 1999.

9. Weiss RA, Feied CF, Weiss MA. Vein Diagnosis and Treatment. New York: McGraw-Hill, 2001.

10. Davis LT, Duffy DM. Determination of incidence and risk factors for postsclerotherapy telangiectatic matting of the lower extremity: a retrospective analysis. J Dermatol Surg Oncol 1990; 16: 327–30.

11. Vin F, Allgert FA, Levardon M. Influence of estrogens and progesterone on the venous system of the lower limbs in women. J Dermatol Surg Oncol 1992; 18: 888–92.

12. Sadick NS. Sclerotherapy of varicose and telangiectatic leg veins. Minimal sclerosant concentrations of hypertonic saline and its relationship to vessel diameter. J Dermatol Surg Oncol 1991; 17: 65–70.

13. McCoy S, Evans A, Spurrier N. Sclerotherapy for leg telangiectasia – a blinded comparative trial of polidocanol and hypertonic saline. Dermatol Surg 1999; 25: 381–6.

14. deFaria JL, Moraes IN. Histopathology of telangiectasias associated with varicose veins. Dermatologica 1963; 127: 321–9.

15. Goldman MP, Weiss RA, Bergan JJ. Varicose Veins and Telangiectasias: Diagnosis and Treatment, 2nd edn. St. Louis, MO: Quality Medical Publishing, 1999.

16. Zimmet S. The prevention of cutaneous necrosis following extravasation of hypertonic saline and sodium tetradecyl sulfate. J Dermatol Surg Oncol 1993; 19: 641–6.

17. Zimmet S. Hyaluronidase in the prevention of sclerotherapy-induced extravasation necrosis: a dose-response study. Dermatol Surg 1996; 22: 73–7.

18. Dorr RT, Alberts DS. Vinca alkaloid skin toxicity: antidote and drug disposition studies in the mouse. J Natl Cancer Inst 1985; 74: 113–20.

19. Campbell CA, Przyklenk K, Kloner RA. Infarct size reduction: a review of the clinical trials. J Clin Pharmacol 1986; 26: 317–29.

20. Mouton RN, Nae M, Otten KT, et al. Morbidity in superficial thrombophlebitis and its potential surgical prevention. Swiss Surg 2003; 9: 15–17.

21. Krause U, Kock HJ, Kroger K, et al. Prevention of deep venous thrombosis associated with superficial thrombophlebitis of the leg by early saphenous vein ligation. Vasa 1998; 27: 34–38.

22. Feied CF. Deep vein thrombosis: the risks of sclerotherapy in hypercoagulable states. Semin Dermatol 1993; 12: 135–49.

23. Conrad P, Malouf GM. The Australian polidocanol open clinical trial results at two years. 7th Annual North American Society of Phlebology Congress, Maui, HI, 1994.

24. Tizes R. Cardiac arrest following routine venipuncture. JAMA 1976; 236: 1846–7.

25. Fisher DA. Treatment of vasovagal reaction. J Am Acad Dermatol 1998; 38: 287–8.

26. Drain KL, Volcheck GW. Preventing and managing drug-induced anaphylaxis. Drug Saf 2001; 24: 843–53.

27. Lieberman P. Anaphylaxis: guidelines for prevention and management. J Respir Dis 1995; 16: 456–62.

28. Levy JH, Roizen MF, Morris JM. Anaphylactic and anaphylactoid reactions: a review. Spine 1986; 11: 282–91.

29. Kanter A, Isaacs M, Gardner M. Ultrasonographically demonstrable AVA in saphenous trunk disease. 6th Annual North American Society of Phlebology Congress, Orlando, FL, 1993.

30. Biegeleisen K, Neilsen RD, O'Shaughnessy A. Inadvertent intraarterial injection complicating ordinary and ultrasound-guided sclerotherapy. J Dermatol Surg Oncol 1993; 19: 953–8.

31. Sternbergh WC, Makhoul RG, Adelman B. Heparin prevents postischemic endothelial cell dysfunction by a mechanism independent of its anticoagulant activity. J Vasc Surg 1993; 17: 318–27.

32. Lazarus HM, Hutto W, Ellertson DG. Therapeutic prevention of ischemia following intraarterial barbiturate injection. J Surg Res 1977; 22: 46–53.

33. Fegan WG, Pegum JM. Accidental intra-arterial injection during sclerotherapy of varicose veins. Br J Surg 1974; 61: 124–6.

34. Bounameaus H, Schneider PA, Huber-Sauteur E, Jolliet PH. Severe ischemia of the hand following intra-arterial promazine injection: effects of vasodilation, anticoagulation, and local thrombolysis with tissue-type plasminogen activator. Vasa 1990; 19: 68–71.

35. Andreev A, Kavrakov T, Petkov D, Penkov P. Severe acute hand ischemia following an accidental intraarterial drug injection, successfully treated with thrombolysis and intraarterial iloprost infusion. Angiology 1995; 10: 963–7.

36. MacGowan WAL, Holland PDJ, Browne HI, Byrnes DP. The local effects of intra-arterial injections of sodium tetradecyl sulphate (S.T.D.) 3 per cent. Br J Surg 1972; 59: 101–4.

37. Bergan JJ, Weiss RA, Goldman MP, Extensive tissue necrosis following high-concentration sclerotherapy for varicose veins. Dermatol Surg 2000; 26: 535–41.

38. Goldman MP, Bergan JL, Guex JJ. Pathophysiology of varicose veins. In: Sclerotherapy: Treatment of Varicose and Telangiectatic Leg Veins, 4th edn. St Louis, MO: Mosby, 2007: Chap 3.

For those contemplating treating hemoglobin-containing structures using light energy, several lasers must be considered. It is inherently more difficult to get photons safely and in sufficient number through melanin into the target chromophore hemoglobin than it is to directly inject a sclerosant into the vessel. The other important issue is that by treating only small superficial vessels, hydrostatic pressure from reverse flow of reflux in larger vessels associated with the telangiectasias is not addressed. For this reason, most laser or intense pulsed light sources are not yet a substitute for sclerotherapy. The depth of penetration of most commonly available wavelengths is insufficient to treat veins that influence hydrostatic pressure.

The reason that light is pursued as an alternative method of chemical irritation, despite these inherent limitations, is that some believe that vaporization of the targeted vessel by complete heating will present minimal inflammatory response compared with chemical irritation of the vessel wall through sclerotherapy. This is theoretical and so far has not been proven. Certainly for superficial facial vessels, particularly those too small to inject, lasers or intense pulsed light have a distinct advantage. Most light-based devices work well for this application. When applied to the legs, however, difficulties arise due to the fact that the overlying skin is thicker, causing greater scatter, and that targeted vessels are of multiple sizes and depths.

When trying to comprehend the vast array of lasers available for the treatment of leg veins, the best starting point is wavelength. Once wavelength is understood in terms of depth of penetration and melanin interaction, the manipulation of that wavelength by pulse duration (width), spot size, fluence, synchronization of pulses, or interval between pulses makes much more sense. Starting with the first laser utilized on blood vessels, the principle of selective photothermolysis was invoked. Selective photothermolysis is based on the fact that the target can absorb certain wavelengths more than the surrounding structures, with a typically short-duration pulse, so that the vessel is destroyed (thermally coagulated) without dissipating heat to surrounding structures and destroying them.

It is known that blue and red veins located in the lower extremities have different clinical and pathophysiologic characteristics that may be associated with the Tyndall effect, vessel depth and size, as well as the degree of oxygenated versus deoxygenated blood content. Because of these circumstances, a novel approach has been adapted to target both red and blue vessels. Shorter wavelengths ranging from 500 to 600 nm have been found to be effective in treating class I oxygenated reddish telangiectasias. Longer wavelengths ranging from 800 to 1100 nm have been shown to be effective in the treatment of class II–III deoxygenated bluish venulectasias and reticular veins.

The wavelength, energy fluence, and pulse duration of light exposure are typically chosen based on the type and size of target vessel being treated. Deeper vessels require a longer wavelength to allow penetration. However, large diameter vessels also require a longer pulse duration to effectively thermocoagulate the entire vessel diameter from front to back wall, this principle being called thermokinetic selectivity. Optimal pulse durations have been calculated for various diameter blood vessels. It is best to examine each laser proceeding from lowest to highest wavelength.

KTP and frequency-doubled Nd:YAG (532 nm)

Modulated krypton triphosphate (KTP) lasers have been reported to be effective at removing leg telangiectasias using pulse durations between 1 and 50 ms. The 532 nm wavelength corresponds to one of several hemoglobin absorption peaks. Although this wavelength does not penetrate deeply into the dermis (about 0.75 mm) relatively specific damage may occur in the vascular target by selecting optimal pulse duration, enlarging the spot size compared an argon laser. Epidermal cooling may allow this wavelength to be more effective.

The most successful outcomes have been achieved in treating vessels with a 1 mm projected spot. This 1 mm spot is advanced 1 mm per pulse, allowing vessels to be traced at 5–10 mm/s. Immediately following laser exposure, the epidermis overlying the vessel appears blanched. Lengthening the pulse duration to match the diameter of the vessel may optimize treatment. A long pulse 532 nm laser (frequency-doubled neodymium-doped yttrium aluminum garnet (Nd:YAG); Versapulse, Coherent, Inc., Palo Alto, CA) has been reported to be somewhat effective in treating leg veins less than 1 mm in diameter that are not directly connected to a feeding reticular vein. With the new Help-G circuitry, along with a 4 °C chilled tip, fluences of 12–20 J/cm² are delivered with a 3–5 mm diameter spot. The pulses are delivered sequentially as the tip glides over water-based gel placed on the skin. Usually, only one pass is necessary to clearly visualize vessel

47

spasm or thrombosis. This is followed within minutes by an urticarial flare around the treated vessels. Some overlying epidermal scabbing may be noted, with hypopigmentation most commonly seen in dark-skinned or tanned patients. There is considerable variation in results reported by individual physicians. Usually, more than one treatment is necessary for maximal vessel improvement, with rare reports of 100% resolution of the leg vein. We believe that the laser is best used for vessels recalcitrant to other laser, intense pulsed light, and sclerotherapy treatment. The use of longer-duration pulses with higher fluence makes this device far more useful for leg veins.

FLPDL (585 nm)

The flashlamp-pulsed dye laser (FLPDL) has been demonstrated to be highly efficacious in treating cutaneous vascular lesions consisting of very small vessels, including port wine stains (PWS), hemangiomas, and facial telangiectasias. The depth of vascular damage is estimated to be 1.5 mm at 585 nm. Therefore, penetration to the typical depth of leg telangiectasias may be achieved. However, telangiectasias over the lower extremities have not responded as well, with less lightening and more post-therapy hyperpigmentation. This may be due to the larger diameter of leg telangiectasias as compared with dermal vessels in PWS. The pulse duration of first-generation FLPDLs was 450 ms, optimal for the 50–100 μm diameter of PWS vessels. This pulse duration is only effective for treating leg telangiectasias less than 0.5 mm in diameter. Many studies have failed to demonstrate satisfactory efficacy. We believe that this is due to failure to recognize the importance of high-pressure vascular flow from feeding reticular and varicose veins and the inherent limitations of a relatively short pulse width. Polla et al treated 35 superficial leg telangiectasias with the FLPDL. The exact laser parameters were not given, except that vessels were treated an average of 2.1 times with a maximum of 4 separate treatments. These vessels were described as being either red–purple and raised, or blue and flat. No mention was made regarding the association of reticular or varicose veins or vessel diameter. Fifteen percent of treated vessels had greater than 75% clearing, with 73% of treated areas showing little response to treatment. The only lesions that responded at all were red–pink tiny telangiectasias. Almost 50% of the treated patients developed persistent hypo- or hyperpigmentation.

Vessels that should optimally respond to FLPDL treatment are predicted to be red telangiectasias less than 0.2 mm in diameter, particularly those vessels arising as a function of telangiectatic matting post sclerotherapy.

Goldman and Fitzpatrick treated 30 female patients with leg telangiectasias less than 0.2 mm in diameter that were red in color. Of 101 telangiectatic patches, 13 were noted to have an associated reticular "feeding" vein between 2 and 3 mm in diameter, which was not treated. Seven patients with 25 patches of telangiectatic matting after previous sclerotherapy were also treated. Thirty-nine telangiectatic patches, chosen

randomly, were treated with laser energies between 7.0 and 8.0 J/cm² and compressed with a rubber "F" compression pad (STD Pharmaceuticals, Hereford, UK). FLDPL-induced hyperpigmentation completely resolved within 4 months. There were no episodes of cutaneous ulceration, thrombophlebitis, or other complications. However, hypopigmentation occurred in some patients with tanned skin. The laser impact sites usually remained hypopigmented for years, and in many cases this was thought to be permanent. With FLPDL treatment, the most effective fluence appears to be between 7.0 and 8.0 J/cm². With these parameters, approximately 67% of telangiectatic patches completely faded within 4 months.

Long-pulse FLPDL (595 nm)

One study utilizing a 595 nm FLPDL at 1.5 ms found over 50% clearance of leg veins at a fluence of 15 J/cm² and approximately 65% clearance at 18 J/cm². In this limited study of 18 patients, vessels ranging in diameter from 0.6 to 1 mm were treated with an elliptical spot size of 2 mm × 7 mm through a transparent hydrogel-based wound dressing. No adverse sequelae were noted at the 5-month follow-up visit.

Lee and Lask treated 25 women with leg telangiectasia less than 1 mm in diameter with the long-pulse FLPDL. Each patient had four areas treated: two with a wavelength of 595 nm at fluences of 15 or 20 J/cm², and two additional areas with 600 nm at 15 or 20 J/cm², respectively. A maximum of three treatments were performed at 6-week intervals. All patients showed improvement. The 595 nm wavelength at 20 J/cm² gave the best results. Treatment response was variable and unpredictable, with some patients having complete resolution and some only slight improvement. Three patients had superficial scabbing, which resolved without apparent scarring. Most patients experienced purpura and hyperpigmentation, which resolved after several weeks. The reasons for the variable efficacy were not reported.

There have been many reports of positive results using the long-pulse 595 nm laser for the removal of leg telangiectasias. An ultralong-pulse laser has been developed with a pulse width of 4 ms (Cynergy, Cynosure, Chelmsford, MA). The 4 ms pulse duration is created by the summation of two individual laser beams each emitting a 2.4 ms pulse that is delivered to the vessels. Alora et al evaluated the efficacy of the 595 nm long-pulse laser using two pulse durations (1.5 and 4 ms) for the treatment of leg veins. Two groups of patients were selected for treatment with the different pulse durations. Group A comprised 27 patients, all of whom had veins less than 1 mm in diameter. A total of three areas were treated: the first two areas were treated with the 4 ms pulse at fluences of 16 and 20 J/cm², and the third area was treated with a 1.5 ms pulse at fluences of 14–16 J/cm². Group B comprised 13 patients: here the first and second areas were treated with the 4 ms pulse and the third area with a 1.5 ms pulse at fluences of 14–16 J/cm². Results showed that the smaller the vessel diameter, the more effective the treatment. The long-pulse dye laser is most effective in targeting lower extremity veins less than

1.5 mm in diameter. Multiple treatments improve on the results obtained after the first treatment.

LPIR (755 nm)

In order to penetrate more deeply to treat larger vessels and to allow for greater thermal diffusion time, a long-pulse infrared alexandrite (LPIR) laser has been developed to allow pulse durations of 20 ms with a spot size of up to 10 mm, utilizing a wavelength that theoretically may penetrate 2–3 mm. The success of this method in fulfilling the requirements of selective photothermolysis awaits a larger number of treated patients.

Diode lasers

Diode lasers do not require bulky gas containers. Coherent monochromatic light is generated through excitation of small diodes. These devices are therefore lightweight and portable, with a relatively small desktop footprint. Presently limited by small spot size and lack of epidermal cooling devices, judgment of clinical efficacy on leg veins awaits larger clinical trials.

A slightly different design is a diode array at 810 nm. This 9 mm × 9 mm wafer is constructed of multiple overlapping interlocking diodes. The pulse duration and intensity can be varied with this fixed spot size. Preliminary studies on small numbers of patients show efficacy on small superficial blood vessels of the leg.

A new approach for the treatment of leg veins is the utilization of electro-optical synergy (ELOS), with a combination of a diode laser and a radiofrequency (RF) system. The premise of ELOS technology is that optical and RF energies have the potential to act in a synergistic manner to achieve selective thermolysis. Sadick and Trelles investigated the efficacy of the Polaris LV™ (Syneron, Irvine, CA), which is based on combined RF and diode laser (915 nm) for the treatment of leg veins. Fifty patients were enrolled in the study, where they received treatment with this system using a fluence between 60 and 80 J/cm² and a conducted RF energy of 100 J/cm³. Each patient received up to three treatment sessions at 6 to 8 week intervals. The results showed that approximately 25% of patients showed over 50% vessel clearance, and about one-third of patients had 75–100% vessel clearance after physician and self assessments. Biopsies were taken from 20 patients, and histologic evaluation showed signs of coagulation and prominent endothelial degeneration in all treated vessels with minimal complications.

High-intensity pulsed light (IPL)

An alternative to lasers in seeking to maximize efficacy in treating purple leg veins is the high-intensity pulsed light (IPL) source. This device permits sequential rapid pulsing, longer-duration pulses, and penetrating longer wavelengths. Since leg venules are substantially larger and have thicker walls than the

ectatic vessels in PWS and hemangiomas, thermal heat diffusion from absorbed red blood cells must require longer times to effectively damage the vein wall. This has been estimated to be 1–10 ms or more. In addition, leg veins contain primary deoxygenated purple blood, not the highly oxygenated blood contained in the vessels of PWS and hemangiomas. Selective wavelengths for hemoglobin as opposed to oxyhemoglobin include 545 nm and a broad peak between 650 and 800 nm. As leg veins are located deeper in the dermis than telangiectasias, a longer wavelength and/or protection of the epidermis and superficial dermis from thermal damage is necessary for ideal treatment.

Theoretically, a phototherapy device that produces a non-coherent light as a continuous spectrum longer than 550 nm should have some advantages over a single-wavelength laser system. First, both hemoglobin and oxyhemoglobin will absorb at a combination of wavelengths. Second, blood vessels located deeper in the dermis will be affected. Third, thermal absorption by the exposed blood vessels should occur with less overlying epidermal absorption, since the longer wavelengths penetrate deeper and are absorbed less by the epidermis.

Utilizing these theoretical considerations, IPL, emitting in the 515–1000 nm range was used at varying energy fluences (5–90 J/cm²) and various pulse durations (2–25 ms) to treat venectasias 0.4–2.0 mm in diameter. Clinical trials using various parameters with the IPL, including multiple pulses of variable duration, demonstrated efficacy ranging from 75 to 90% total clearance in vessels less than 0.2 mm in diameter, to 80% in vessels of 0.2–0.5 mm diameter, and 80% in vessels of 0.5–1 mm diameter. The incidence of adverse sequelae was minimal, with hypopigmentation occurring in 1–5% of patients and resolving within 4–6 months. Tanned or darkly pigmented patients were likely to develop hypo- and hyperpigmentation in addition to blistering and superficial erosions. These all cleared over a few months. Treatment parameters that were found to be most successful for vessels smaller than 0.3 mm included a single pulse of 22 J/cm² in 3 ms or a double pulse of 35–40 J/cm² given in 2.4 and 4.0 ms with a 10 ms delay. Vessels between 0.2 and 0.5 mm were treated with the same double-pulse parameters or with a 3.0–6.0 ms pulse at 35–40 J/cm² with a 20 ms delay. Vessels larger than 0.5 mm were treated with a triple pulse of 3.5/3.1/2.5 ms with pulse delays of 20 ms at a fluence of 50 J/cm² or with a triple pulse of 3/4/6 ms with pulse delays of 30 ms at a fluence of 55–60 J/cm². The choice of a cut-off filter was based on skin color, with light-skinned patients using a 550 nm filter and darker-skinned patients a 570 or 590 nm filter.

Increased efficacy was achieved by increasing the pulse durations to a maximum of 10 ms in two consecutive pulses separated by a 20 ms delay with a 570 nm cut-off filter and fluences of 75 J/cm². Response rates of 74% were achieved in two treatments with an 8% incidence of temporary hypo- or hyperpigmentation. By combining a shorter pulse (2–4, 5.0 ms) with a longer pulse (7–10 ms), it is theoretically possible to ablate smaller and larger vessels overlying one another in the dermis.

An emerging IPL technology to eliminate vascular lesions on the lower extremities includes Lumenis One (Santa Clara, CA). In a study with 31 patients to remove leg telangiectases, each person received a total of four treatment sessions at up to 5-week intervals. IPL treatments were performed with the 15 mm × 35 mm or 8 mm × 15 mm light guides with 3–100 ms pulses at a broad spectrum (515–1200 nm) with a fluence range of 10–40 J/cm². After the third treatment session, all lesions responded to the delivered treatment and were in remission resulting in significant improvement. Ninety percent of patients reported that they were very satisfied to extremely satisfied after the three treatments.

A new IPL technology that has emerged has the capability of a variable pulse width and fluence and includes an integrated optimal skin cooling system (Starlux, Palomar Medical Technologies, Inc., Burlington, MA). The laser can be utilized in various procedures, including the treatment of leg veins, delivering fluences up to 700 J/cm² for powerful vein clearance. Mordon et al evaluated the efficacy of the IPL/1064 nm system on the reduction of 1–2 mm blue telangiectasias on the leg. Eighteen patients received two or three treatment sessions using a fluence between 300 and 360 J/cm² and a spot size of 2 mm on the treatment area. The results showed that 55% of vessels treated were cleared after one treatment session, 86% after two sessions, and 98% after three sessions. No anesthesia was needed for the treatments. Adverse events included moderate pain, mild erythema, edema, hyperpigmentation, and matting.

Other studies and treatments have looked at the effect of combination of the Nd:YAG laser and IPL for the treatment of leg veins. A group of 38 patients were treated for deep (up to 5 mm) and large (up to 3 mm in diameter) reticular veins. A reduction of the venous network of 80–90% after two treatment sessions with the Nd:YAG laser was obtained in 84% of patients. Three successive treatment sessions with IPL achieved complete vanishing of the treated venous network in 36 of the 38 patients. These results show that the combined action of Nd:YAG laser and IPL can be effective in the treatment of deep and extensive reticular networks of the lower extremity.

Treatment of leg telangiectasias can be accomplished with IPL. A variety of parameters have been shown to be effective. Testing a few different parameters during the first treatment session and using the most efficient and least painful parameter on subsequent treatments is recommended. This trend towards a combination approach using IPL technology with lasers has resulted in improved results and patient satisfaction in removing leg veins.

Near-infrared 1064 nm laser

The Nd:YAG laser at 1064 nm is also used to treat leg telangiectasias. The average depth of penetration in human skin is 0.75 mm and a reduction to 10% of incident power occurs at a depth of 3.7 mm. Thus, this laser is well suited to treat blood vessels within the mid dermis. The 1064 nm wavelength is absorbed by water, to some degree by hemoglobin, and to a far lesser degree by melanin.

At this wavelength, melanin has minimal influence on absorption. The 1064 nm wavelength allows darker skin types to be treated with minimal risks to the epidermis due to decreased interaction with hemoglobin. The main light-absorbing chromophore filling a vessel is hemoglobin. As previously stated, it has a broad band of absorption from 800 to 1100 nm. Dermal transmission of these wavelengths due to less scatter at 1064 nm allows penetration into the depth of a dermal blood vessel. Theoretically, incomplete absorption by hemoglobin itself allows full-thickness vessel penetration. This penetration permits better treatment of vessels larger than 1 mm and up to 3–4 mm deep. Most telangiectatic webs of the leg consist of multiple-size vessels from 0.5 to 2 mm, including larger blue reticular veins of 3 mm, all of which can be treated with the 1064 nm wavelength laser. Clinical results with a new multiple synchronized pulsed 1064 nm laser indicate that this longer wavelength supplied at pulses of up to 16 ms appears to be a valuable modality for immediate closure and subsequent elimination of leg telangiectasias.

Omura et al evaluated the effectiveness of a single treatment with a 1064 nm Nd:YAG laser (Coolglide, Cutera, Brisbane, CA) in the treatment of reticular veins in the lower extremity. Twenty patients with reticular veins ranging from 1 to 3 mm in diameter received one treatment with the Nd:YAG laser at a fluence of 100 J/cm² and a 50 ms pulse duration. The results showed that two-thirds of vessels cleared more than 75% at 1 and 3 months after treatment. Larger vessels responded more effectively than smaller vessels. Minimal side-effects included superficial thrombosis, delayed bruising, hyperpigmentation, and matting.

Sadick addressed the efficacy of a high-power 50 ms 1064 nm Nd:YAG laser (Lyra, Laserscope, San Jose, CA). Each of 10 patients with 5 cm² area of veins measuring 0.2–3 mm in diameter received up to three treatment sessions. Red and blue vessels were treated in a similar manner with fluences in the ranges 250–370 J/cm² (blue veins) and 400–600 J/cm² (red veins) and pulse widths of 30–50 ms (red veins) and 50–60 ms (blue veins). Three months after the last treatment session, 20% of the vessels treated showed 50–75% improvement, with equal clearing of red and blue vessels, while at 6 months, 80% of patients displayed 75% or greater improvement. Nine of the 10 patients were highly satisfied with the treatment. Side-effects included bruising, hyperpigmentation, and blistering/crusting, where all cases were resolved. Another study conducted by Sadick examined the effectiveness of a different 1064 nm Nd:YAG laser for the treatment of leg veins (Gemini, Laserscope, San Jose, CA). Fifty female patients (mean age 37 years) with class I–III red telangiectasias, blue venulectasias, and reticular veins (0.1–4.0 mm in diameter) on the inner or outer thighs were treated. A combined approach of laser/IPL treatment was used; patients had up to three treatments at 6-week intervals on a 5 cm² surface area, with the use of an IPL source wavelength of 550 nm and a fluence of 40 J/cm² for treatment of red telangiectases less than 1 mm in diameter, while a 1064 nm Nd:YAG laser at a fluence of

140 J/cm^2 was used to treat venulectasias and reticular vessels that were 1.0–4.0 mm in diameter. Two to three treatment sessions produced significant clearing (75–100%) of veins in 80% of patients. The mean erythema index showed significant lightening (35.3+dl) in the study population for the treated area. Seventy-six percent of patients reported great satisfaction with the treatment results. A bimodal wavelength approach utilizing both short and long wavelengths appears to produce significant clearing of the variably colored, multiple-diameter/depth array of vessels with both patients and physicians being satisfied with the treatment results.

Goldman and Fitzpatrick also studied the effect of combined sclerotherapy/laser treatment. Twenty-seven patients had either bilaterally symmetrical telangiectatic patches or a large "sunburst" telangiectatic flare, which could be divided into two separate treatment sites. Patients were treated at one site with the FLPDL alone, or with laser fluences 1–2 J/cm^2 less than that utilized with FLPDL alone immediately before injection of the telangiectasias with polidocanol (POL), 0.25%, 0.5%, or 0.75%, with a volume of 0.1–0.25 mL per injection site.

Forty-four percent of combination-treated areas completely resolved. There appeared to be little difference in efficacy and adverse sequelae with concentrations of POL between 0.25% and 0.75%. There did appear to be greater improvement with laser energies of 7.5–7.75 J/cm^2. As with the FLPDL alone, treatment site did not appear to significantly affect outcome, except for an increased incidence of complications in the ankle and knee areas.

The most significant difference between the FLPDL alone and combination treatment was the incidence of complications. With combination treatment, post-treatment ulceration and telangiectatic matting occurred in 11% of treated areas, compared with 0% using FLPDL alone. Of 23 non-ulcerated treatment sites, 6 developed persistent pigmentation beyond 1 year. Of 27 sites, 2 developed telangiectatic matting, which lasted over 1 year. Of 27 treatment sites, 4 developed superficial ulceration. In these ulcerated patients, laser fluences were at least 6.5 J/cm^2 and POL concentration was at least 0.5%.

In conclusion, FLPDL when pulsed at 450 μs is an effective modality for treating red leg telangiectasias up to 0.2 mm in diameter. FLPDL treatment is efficacious for both essential telangiectasias and vessels of telangiectatic matting. This form of treatment alone has a low incidence of complications. The optimal laser fluence is between 7.0 and 8.0 J/cm^2. Treatment is most effective if all vessels larger than 0.2 mm in diameter, especially varicose and reticular feeding veins, are treated first with sclerotherapy or another modality. Results are not affected by vessel location. Post-treatment compression of such small vessels (<0.2 mm) appears unnecessary. Combination treatment appears to offer no advantage to laser alone and appears to have a significant degree of complica-

tions when treatment is limited to red telangiectasias less than 0.2 mm in diameter.

Since sclerotherapy is relatively cost-effective compared with laser or IPL treatment, when is it appropriate to use these latter advanced therapies? Obviously, patients who are needle-phobic may better tolerate laser treatment, even though the pain from the laser is probably greater. In addition, patients who are prone to telangiectatic matting are also appropriate candidates. Vessels below the ankle are particularly appropriate to treat with light, since sclerotherapy has a relatively high incidence of ulceration in this area due to the higher distribution of arteriovenous anastamoses. Patients who have vessels resistant to sclerotherapy are excellent candidates. Seventy-five percent clearance of sclerotherapy-resistant telangiectasias was achieved with two or three treatments of IPL.

We believe that the optimal treatment of leg telangiectasias will utilize sclerotherapy, followed by laser or IPL with a rationale similar to that described above (FLPDL/sclerotherapy). Sclerotherapy will treat the feeding venous system, with laser or IPL effectively sealing superficial vessels to decrease the complications of extravasation of sclerosant and ischemic ulceration with resulting pigmentation, recanalization, ulceration, and telangiectatic matting.

Light- and laser-based technologies play a definite role in the treatment of leg telangiectasias. Smaller vessels can be effectively treated by green (532 nm), yellow (600 nm), and red (794–800 nm) lasers, as well as noncoherent IPL (550–1000 nm) and near-infrared (1064 nm), with each having unique characteristics specific to spot size, pulse duration, and fluence. The most promising new wavelength applied to leg veins is in the infrared range of 1064 nm, raising the possibility of treating larger and deeper vessels with less risk to the epidermis. Use of concomitant sclerotherapy may enhance the results of lasers and IPL alone. The exact role for each device will continue to evolve.

Adrian RM. Treatment of leg telangiectasias using a long-pulse frequency-doubled neodymium:YAG laser at 532 nm. Dermatol Surg 1998; 24: 19–23.

Anderson RR, Parrish JA. The optics of human skin. J Invest Dermatol 1981; 77: 13–19.

Apfelberg DB, Smith T, Maser MR, et al. Study of three laser systems for treatment of superficial varicosities of the lower extremity. Lasers Surg Med 1987; 7: 219–23.

Ashton N. Corneal vascularization. In: Duke-Elder S, Perkins ES, eds. The Transparency of the Cornea. Oxford: Blackwell, 1960.

Chess C, Chess Q. Cool laser optics treatment of large telangiectasia of the lower extremities. J Dermatol Surg Oncol 1993; 19: 74–80.

Colaiuda S, Colaiuda F, Gasparotti M. Treatment of deep under-lying reticular veins by Nd:Yag laser and IPL source. Minerva Cardioangiol 2000; 48: 329–34.

Corcos L, Longo L. Classification and treatment of telangiectases of the lower limbs. Laser 1988; 1: 22–7.

Dixon JA, Rotering RH, Huethner SE. Patient's evaluation of argon laser therapy of port-wine stain, decorative tattoos, and essential telangiectasia. Lasers Surg Med 1984; 4: 181–90.

Dvorak HF. Tumors: wounds that do not heal: similarities between tumor stroma generation and wound healing. N Engl J Med 1986; 315: 1650–9.

Folkman J, Klagsbrun M. Angiogenic factors. Science 1987; 235: 442–7.

Garden JM, Tan OT, Kerschmann R, et al. Effect of dye laser pulse duration on selective cutaneous vascular injury. J Invest Dermatol 1986; 87: 653–7.

Goldman MP, Eckhouse S. Photothermal sclerosis of leg veins. ESC Medical Systems, LTD Photoderm VL Cooperative Study Group. Dermatol Surg 1996; 22: 323–30.

Goldman MP, Fitzpatrick RE. Cutaneous Laser Surgery: The Art and Science of Selective Photothermolysis, 2nd edn. St Louis, MO: Mosby-Year Book, 1998.

Goldman MP, Fitzpatrick RE. Pulsed-dye laser treatment of leg telangiectasia with and without simultaneous sclerotherapy. J Dermatol Surg Oncol 1990; 16: 338–44.

Goldman MP, Martin DE, Fitzpatrick RE, Ruiz-Esparza J. Pulsed dye laser treatment of telangiectasia with and without subtherapeutic sclerotherapy: clinical and histologic examination in the rabbit ear vein model. J Am Acad Dermatol 1990; 23: 23–30.

Hsia J, Lowery JA, Zelickson B. Treatment of leg telangiectasia using a long-pulse dye laser at 595 nm. Lasers Surg Med 1997; 20: 1–5.

Lee PK, Lask GP. Treatment of leg veins by long pulse dye laser (Sclerolaser). Lasers Surg Med 1997; Suppl 9: 40.

Majewski S, Kaminski M, Jablonska S, et al. Angiogenic capability of peripheral blood mononuclear cells in psoriasis. Arch Dermatol 1985; 121: 1018–21.

Mordon S, Brisot D, Fournier N. Using a "non uniform pulse sequence" can improve selective coagulation with a Nd:YAG laser (1.06 µm) thanks to met-hemoglobin absorption: a clinical study on blue leg veins. Lasers Surg Med 2003; 32: 160–70.

Nakagawa H, Tan OT, Parrish JA. Ultrastructural changes in human skin after exposure to a pulsed laser. J Invest Dermatol 1985; 84: 396–400.

Omura NE, Dover JS, Arndt KA, Kauvar AN. Treatment of reticular leg veins with a 1064 nm long pulsed Nd:YAG laser. J Am Acad Dermatol 2003; 48: 76:81.

Polla LL, Tan OT, Garden JM, Parrish JA. Tunable pulsed dye laser for the treatment of benign cutaneous vascular ectasia. Dermatologica 1987; 174: 11–17.

Railan D, Parlette EC, Uebelhoer NS, Rohrer TE. Laser treatment of vascular lesions. Clin Dermatol 2005; 24: 8–15.

Raulin C, Weiss RA, Schonermark MP. Treatment of essential telangiectasias with an intense pulsed light source (PhotoDerm VL). Dermatol Surg 1997; 23: 941–6.

Ryan TJ. Factors influencing the growth of vascular endothelium in the skin. Br J Dermatol 1970; 82(Suppl 5): 99.

Sadick NS. A dual wavelength approach for laser/intense pulsed light source treatment of lower extremity veins. J Am Acad Dermatol 2002; 46: 66–72.

Sadick NS, Weiss RA, Goldman MP. Advances in laser surgery for leg veins: bimodal wavelength approach to lower extremity vessels, new cooling techniques, and longer pulse durations. Dermatol Surg 2002; 28: 16–20.

Sadick NS. Laser treatment with a 1064 nm laser for lower extremity class I–III veins employing variable spots and pulse width parameters. Dermatol Surg 2003; 29: 916–19.

Sadick NS, Trelles M. A clinical histological, and computer based assessment of the Polaris LV, combination diode, and radiofrequency system, for leg vein treatment. Lasers Surg Med 2005; 36: 98–104.

Schroeter CA, Wilder D, Reineke T, et al. Clinical significance of an intense, pulsed light source on leg telangiectasias of up to 1 mm diameter. Eur J Dermatol 1997; 7: 38–42.

Sherwood KA, Murray S, Kurban AK, Tan OT. Effect of wavelength on cutaneous pigment using pulsed irradiation. J Invest Dermatol 1989; 92: 717–20.

Tan OT, Carney JM, Margolis R, et al. Histologic responses of port-wine stains treated by argon, carbon dioxide, and tunable dye lasers: a preliminary report. Arch Dermatol 1986; 122: 1016–22.

Tan OT, Kerschmann R, Parrish JA. Effect of skin temperature on selective vascular injury caused by pulsed laser irradiation. J Invest Dermatol 1985; 85: 441–4.

Weiss RA, Weiss MA. Photothermal sclerosis of resistant telangiectatic leg and facial veins using the PhotoDerm VL. Annual Meeting of the Mexican Academy of Dermatology, Monterey, Mexico, April 24, 1996.

Weiss RA, Weiss MA. Intense pulsed light revisited: progressive increase in pulse durations for better results on leg veins. 11th Annual North American Society of Phlebology Congress, Palm Desert, CA, November, 1997.

Weiss RA, Weiss MA. Combination intense pulsed light and sclerotherapy — a synergistic effect. 11th Annual North American Society of Phlebology Congress, Palm Desert, CA, November 1997.

Zamir B. Lumenis One — an expandable technology platform for comprehensive aesthetic treatments. White Paper 2004; 1–8.

Zelickson BD, Mehregan DA, Zarrin AA, et al. Clinical, histologic, and ultrastructural evaluation of tattoos treated with three laser systems. Lasers Surg Med 1994; 15: 364–72.

Introduction

Great saphenous vein (GSV) reflux is the most common underlying cause of significant varicose veins. The most durable treatment has historically been surgical ligation and stripping. Although frequently successful in eliminating the pathophysiologic superficial venous hypertension and unsightly varicose veins, this procedure, usually requiring general anesthesia, has been associated with a high incidence of perioperative morbidity and significant varicose vein recurrence. In an attempt to diminish morbidity, lesser surgical treatments such as high ligation of the GSV at the saphenofemoral junction (SFJ) (crossectomy) were employed; unfortunately, even in combination with phlebectomy of varicose tributaries, this usually resulted in recurrence of varicose veins soon thereafter. As duplex ultrasound technology improved, the potential for even less invasive, image guided therapies was harnessed. In 1998, radiofrequency (RF) thermal ablation of the great saphenous vein by a novel endoluminal approach was carried out by several European centers. The following year, laser energy was used to produce a similar thermal injury to the endothelium. Thermal treatment with either method results in contraction of vein wall collagen and/or iterative obliteration of the vessel lumen. Thermal ablation, having been used to treat hundreds of thousands of patients in the last decade with excellent short- and long term results, should now be accepted as the treatment of choice for insufficiency of both the truncal GSV and small saphenous vein (SSV), as well as a variety of other incompetent superficial tributary and perforating veins.

Radiofrequency ablation

Endovenous RF ablation (RFA), also called the VNUS Closure procedure, is a minimally invasive alternative to vein stripping for elimination of saphenous vein reflux. The main feature of the technology is the precise application of RF energy via a catheter that is placed endoluminally to deliver heat to the vein wall, resulting in vein shrinkage or occlusion by contraction of venous wall collagen. The current ClosurePlus™ and ClosureRFS™ catheters accomplish this by the principle of resistive heating using bipolar electrodes in contact with the vein wall. The catheter design includes collapsible catheter electrodes around which the vein may shrink

and a central lumen to allow a guidewire and/or fluid delivery within the 6F catheter. A larger 8F catheter allows treatment of saphenous veins upwards of 24 mm in diameter. The ClosureRFS™ catheter employs a pair of fixed diameter electrodes. All of these catheters utilize a feedback mechanism from a thermocouple in the vicinity of the electrodes or heating element. By limiting temperature to 85–90°C, thermal injury is confined to the vein endothelium, media, and close perivenous vicinity, typically 1–2 mm. Electrode mediated RF vein wall ablation is a self limiting process. As coagulation of tissue occurs, there is a marked decrease in impedance that limits heat generation. Alternatively, if clot builds up on the electrodes, blood is heated instead of tissue and there is a marked rise in impedance (resistance to RF). The RF generator can be programmed to rapidly shut down when impedance rises, thus assuring minimal heating of blood but efficient heating of the vein wall.

Method (Figure 10.1)

The patient is placed in a supine position on an adjustable table for the procedure. Some practitioners elect to provide oral or intravenous sedation. The course of the GSV from the SFJ to near the knee is mapped and marked with indelible ink. A patch of nitroglycerin paste on paper tape may be applied to the opposed insertion site prior to the venous surgical prep to help dilate the vein and prevent venospasm that would make percutaneous access difficult. The leg is circumferentially cleansed, groin-to-ankle, with antiseptic. Sterile Stockinet is often used to cover the foot, ankle, and distal calf. A split sheet drape is used to isolate the leg. After infiltration of local anesthetic to the insertion site, under ultrasound guidance, the GSV is accessed with a 19 or 21 gauge needle. Using the Seldinger technique, the introducer sheath is advanced into the vein. A radiofrequency Closure catheter is advanced, under ultrasound guidance, up to just below the entrance of the superficial epigastric vein and/or is confluent with the SFJ. This position is confirmed by ultrasound. Approximately 200 ml of 0.1% lidocaine or another dilute local anesthetic is then injected directly, under ultrasound guidance, into the saphenous compartment from the insertion site up to 1 cm below the SFJ. This solution provides the local anesthetic, protects the surrounding tissues from heat related damage, and compresses the vein around the catheter electrodes, ensuring complete vein wall treatment. The patient is placed in a moderate Trendelenburg

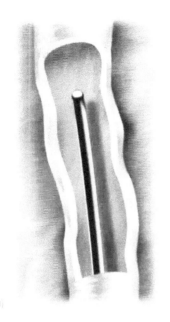 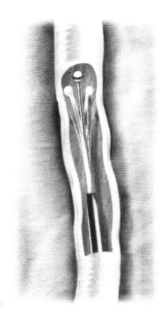 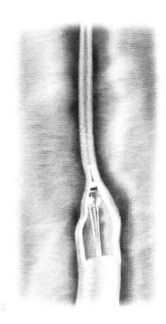

(a) ClosurePlus™ catheter advanced to furthest treatment site. (b) Electrodes deployed, radiofrequency energy initiated. (c) Catheter withdrawn, closing vein. (Illustration courtesy and copyright of VNUS Medical Technologies, Inc., San Jose, CA)

position and the final position of the catheter tip is confirmed by ultrasound. External compression is applied to the leg over the catheter tip as it is withdrawn. The withdrawal rate is adjusted to maintain the temperature of the tip at 85–90°C. On conclusion of the procedure, patency of the common femoral artery and vein, as well as successful contraction of the GSV with a residual diameter of less than 2 mm, are confirmed by duplex examination. Patients are then placed in short-stretch bandages and 30–40 mmHg graduated compression stockings and instructed to walk at least 30 minutes per day, use elevation and intermittent ice on the treated portion of the leg for 24–48 hours, and to otherwise resume normal activity immediately. They are told to avoid weight lifting, but resumption of aerobic exercise is encouraged.

Results

The validity and efficacy of the original Closure procedure has been borne out by numerous published reports. Of 1222 veins treated with 85°C from 34 centers worldwide, vein occlusion rates were between 85.5% and 88.3%, and reflux-free rates were between 53.3% and 88.2% at annual follow-up out to 5 years. Efficacy at 1–2 years was reported to be between 92% and 97% in other published studies. Clinical symptom improvement, measured by absence of limb pain, fatigue or edema, was observed in 85–94% of limbs classified as having anatomic success at annual intervals over the 5-year period. Clinical improvement was also observed in 70–80% of limbs in the anatomic failure group. Several prospective randomized studies comparing Closure treatment with vein stripping and ligation showed significant clinical superiority of the Closure procedure in terms of postoperative pain, patient recovery, and patient quality of life.

RFA – additional considerations

In addition to GSV ablation, the Closure procedure has been extended to treat the SSV and accessory saphenous veins with similarly excellent results. In the case of SSV treatment, careful ultrasound guidance is critical for precise placement of the catheter electrodes to avoid inadvertent heating of the posterior tibial nerve. Pain located in the heel or foot at onset of heating indicates placement too close to the nerve. Tumescent anesthesia infiltrated circumferentially around the SSV is also critical to avoid injury to this nerve or to the sural nerve, which usually lies near the vein in the mid calf.

Endovenous ablation of incompetent perforators can be facilitated by the ClosureRFS™ and ClosureRFSflex™ devices (Figure 10.2). Incompetent perforators have been traditionally treated by surgical ligation or subfascial endoscopic perforator surgery (SEPS). SEPS is less invasive than traditional surgery, but has limitations such as its inability to access certain perforator veins, relatively complex technology, significant long-term recurrence rate, difficulty associated with repeat treatment, and its requirement of general anesthesia. Using the ClosureRFS™ procedure, the vessel is accessed directly, using ultrasound guidance, and requires only local anesthesia without epinephrine. Treatment is accomplished by delivering RF energy over a short segment at the subfascial level (Figure 10.3). The perforator that is incompetent can be targeted, and, if necessary, repeat treatment can be easily performed. Small tributary and accessory saphenous veins can also be treated with these devices.

The advantage of RFA over other endovenous thermal ablation techniques is that the energy delivery is controlled by the temperature sensor on the catheter, thus minimizing vessel perforation and its associated postoperative pain and bruising.

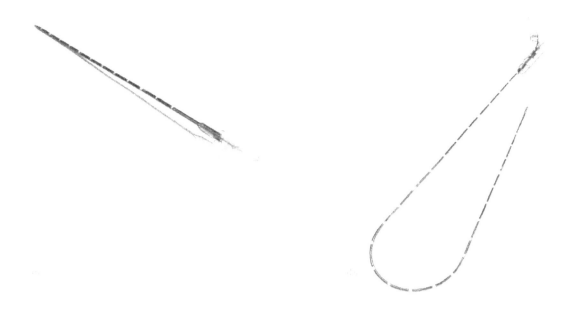

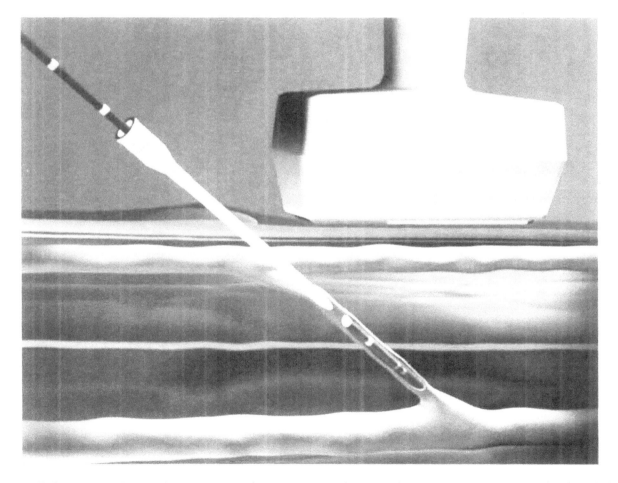

A disadvantage has been the relatively long procedure time required to satisfactorily ablate the vein segment. Most recently, a new generation of Closure catheter, ClosureFAST™ (Figure 10.4), has been developed to substantially shorten the procedure time. The new catheter employs a 7 cm heating element that heats to 120°C through conductive heating, equating to tissue temperatures in the range 100–110°C. A temperature sensor is located on the heating element to control the treatment temperature and power, and to provide feedback on the adequacy of exsanguination and compression. The catheter remains stationary during a 20 s energy delivery period. It is then repeatedly retracted 6.5 cm, guided by shaft markers, and energized for 20 s at each segment until the desired length of vein has been treated. Additional 20 s cycles can be delivered for segments of larger diameter.

The ClosureFAST™ catheter has undergone successful early clinical studies. In a series of 252 limbs treated, initially presented by Proebstle, the average energy delivery time was 2.2 minutes over an average 37 cm vein length and the average procedure time from catheter insertion to final removal was 16.6 minutes. Initial vein occlusion was 100%, and all veins examined at up to 6 months follow-up remained closed. Careful placement of the catheter tip, verified by ultrasound, approximately 2 cm distal to the junction with the deep vein is an absolute necessity to avoid injury to the deep system and minimize the potential for subsequent deep vein thrombosis (DVT).

Laser ablation

In 1999, Boné first reported on delivery of endoluminal laser energy. Since then, a method for treating the entire incompetent GSV segment has been described. Endovenous laser treatment, which received approval from the US Food and Drug Administration (FDA) in January 2002, creates vein

occlusion by delivery of laser energy directly into the vein walls via a bare-tipped laser fiber (Figure 10.5). Lasers with wavelengths of 810, 940, 980, and 1320 nm have all been used with reported success. Maximal contact between the laser and the vein wall is necessary to cause sufficient damage to the vein, resulting in vein wall thickening with eventual contraction and fibrosis.

Method

Subjects with varicose veins due to incompetence of the GSV, SSV, anterior accessory GSV (ASV), or other incompetent veins may be candidates for endovenous laser. Duplex ultrasound is used to mark the skin overlying the incompetent portion of the target vein, starting at the highest point of reflux, and a percutaneous entry point is chosen. In almost all cases, the target vein is entered directly, although access may be gained via one of its direct tributaries. Entry via a tributary

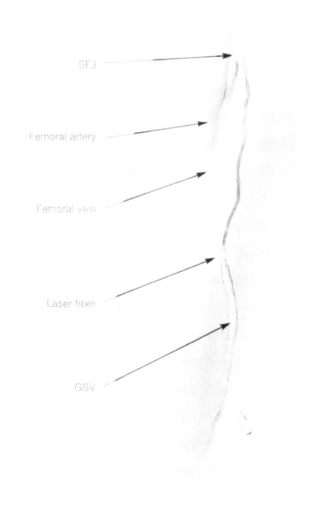

SFJ

Femoral artery

Femoral vein

Laser fiber

GSV

Endovenous laser treatment of the great saphenous vein (GSV). Laser energy is delivered to the inner walls of the GSV as the laser fiber is withdrawn from the saphenofemoral junction (SFJ) to the entry site, resulting in contraction of the vein. (Illustration courtesy and copyright of Diomed, Inc., Andover, MD)

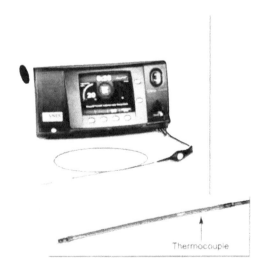

Thermocouple

VNUS ClosureFAST™ catheter. (Image courtesy and copyright of VNUS Medical Technologies, Inc., San Jose, CA)

should only be attempted if the vein is relatively straight and of sufficient diameter, since these veins tend to be more prone to venospasm and can be more difficult to traverse. In general, the vein is punctured at or just distal to the lowest level of reflux as determined by duplex ultrasound.

Using local anesthesia and ultrasound guidance, the target vein is punctured and a 5F vascular sheath with centimeter markings is inserted over a guidewire into the vein and passed proximally through the entire abnormal segment and into a more central vein (femoral vein when treating GSV, popliteal vein when treating SSV, and GSV when treating a GSV tributary). A bare-tipped laser fiber is inserted into the sheath and passed to a point more proximal than the expected final position. The sheath is then pulled back, exposing the tip of the fiber, and the fiber is locked in place. Using ultrasound guidance, the sheath and fiber are withdrawn as a unit out of the more central vein and positioned just distal to its junction with the vein to be treated. When treating the GSV, the laser should be placed below the junction of the superficial epigastric vein (Figure 10.6). The fiber is left in this position during tumescent anesthesia administration and is re-positioned just prior to delivery of laser energy.

Tumescent anesthesia should make endovenous laser painless, precluding the need for intravenous sedation or general anesthesia. Proper delivery of the fluid will also maximize safety and efficacy of endovenous laser treatment by ensuring

compression of the entire vein around the laser fiber (Figure 10.7). Inadequate vein emptying will lead to suboptimal vein wall heating. In this case, occlusion may be due to thrombosis, which will inevitably result in recanalization. Many practitioners also believe that the surrounding cuff of tumescent fluid also serves as a protective barrier preventing heating of nontarget tissues.

Injection of tumescent fluid in the proper plane can only be achieved under ultrasound guidance. The tumescent fluid should be delivered between the target vein and adjacent nontarget tissues, preferably by positioning the needle within the saphenous compartment. Anesthetic fluid may be delivered using hand pressure and a 1-inch 25 gauge needle attached to a 20 cm³ syringe, via a refillable syringe connected to an IV bag containing the anesthetic, and by use of an infusion pump.

To treat a 45 cm segment of vein, approximately 100–150 cm³ of 0.1% lidocaine neutralized with sodium bicarbonate may be required. This mixture can be made by diluting 50 cm³ of 1% lidocaine in 450 cm³ of normal saline and adding 10 cm³ of 8.4% sodium bicarbonate. If it is anticipated that larger volumes of tumescent anesthesia will be necessary, a concentration of 0.05% lidocaine can be used effectively. These amounts of lidocaine are well within the safe doses of 4.5 mg/kg of lidocaine without epinephrine and 7 mg/kg with epinephrine.

Proper tumescent anesthesia and Trendelenberg position will facilitate vein emptying and usually result in sufficient laser fiber and vein wall contact. Raising the leg, manual compression, applying suction to the sheath, or cooling the room to induce vasospasm may also help to empty the vein. Since the laser fiber can move during tumescent anesthesia administration, the laser fiber is re-positioned prior to delivery of laser

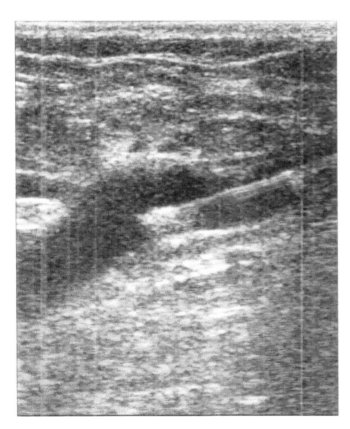

Laser tip in position at the saphenofemoral junction and distal to the superficial epigastric vein. (Image courtesy of Helane S Fronek MD)

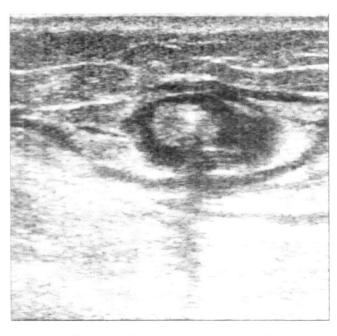

Tumescent fluid surrounds the great saphenous vein. (Image courtesy of Helane S Fronek MD)

energy. Confirmation of the position can also be made by direct visualization of the red aiming beam through the skin. For the GSV, the fiber tip is positioned at or below a competent superficial epigastric vein, or 5–10 mm peripheral to the SFJ. When treating the SSV, seeing the fiber tip can be difficult due to the acute angle taken by the SSV as it dives to join the popliteal vein. Accurate pre-procedure marking of the SPJ is important, and, when used with the red aiming beam, this will enable precise positioning of the laser fiber. Optimally, the laser fiber tip is placed 10–15 mm peripheral to the SPJ where the SSV turns parallel to the skin just below the popliteal fossa, although the exact location of the SPJ is quite variable in different patients.

The marked vascular sheath and fiber are withdrawn together during laser energy delivery, at about 2 mm/s, in order to deliver at least 70 J/cm throughout the treated segment (Figure 10.8). Manual withdrawal also allows laser energy delivery to be customized to the particular vein segment being treated, which enhances treatment efficacy and safety. For example, higher laser energies are delivered to the most central portion of the GSV, with the first 10–15 cm of the vein treated with 140 J/cm, which is achieved by withdrawing the laser fiber at a rate of 1 mm/s. This segment of the GSV is the most prone to treatment failure and is the least susceptible to venospasm. Thus, it is necessary to deliver proportionately larger amounts of tumescent anesthesia and more laser energy to adequately treat this important vein segment.

A class II (30–40 mmHg) graduated support stocking is worn for at least 1–2 weeks at all times except to sleep or to shower. The use of graduated support stockings, in addition to immediate and frequent ambulation, will lower the risk of superficial thrombophlebitis in tributary varices, increase the velocity of blood flow in the deep veins to reduce the likelihood of DVT, and diminish discomfort following the procedure.

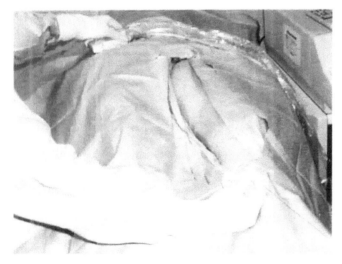

The laser fiber and sheath are withdrawn at a rate of 3 mm/s using 14 W, delivering an average of 70 J/cm to the vein. (Image courtesy of Robert Min)

Patients are followed clinically and with duplex ultrasound examinations performed within 1 week, at the completion of treatment, and yearly thereafter. Compression sclerotherapy or ambulatory phlebectomy treatment of distal varicose tributaries is performed as needed. Duplex ultrasound criteria for successful treatment are the following:

- at 1 week, a noncompressible GSV with echogenic, thickened vein walls, and no flow seen within the occluded vein lumen upon color Doppler interrogation
- at 3–6 months' follow-up, an occluded GSV with substantial (at least 50%) reduction in diameter
- at 1 year and beyond, complete disappearance of the GSV or minimal residual fibrous cord with no flow detectable

Results

In the first 1000 limbs treated with endovenous laser for saphenous vein reflux at Weill Cornell Vascular, using an 810 nm diode laser (Diomed, Inc., Andover, MA), successful endovenous occlusion was seen in 98% of treated limbs (982/1000) at up to 5 years' follow-up. Ninety-nine percent (457/460) of treated vein segments were occluded at over 2 years. The majority (13/18) of failures occurred prior to 1 year. All veins treated with at least 70 J/cm of laser energy have remained closed. Clinical examination correlated well to the duplex ultrasound findings. All subjects demonstrated improvement of visible varicosities (Figure 10.9).

Following successful endovenous laser treatment, all subjects presenting with pain noted resolution or substantial improvement in associated symptoms. Non-puncture site bruising was seen in 24% of limbs at 1-week follow-up. Some patients experienced discomfort over the treated vein beginning hours after the procedure, and many patients also noted a delayed tightness and pulling sensation most likely caused by retraction of the vein. Others have reported similar success rates of endovenous laser ablation of the GSV. These studies have consistently shown successful fibrotic occlusion of the target truncal vein in 90–100% of cases, with very rare recanalization of previously occluded vein segments. Clinical improvement was noted in almost all cases following successful truncal vein occlusion. Patient acceptance was high and adverse reactions, including skin burns, paresthesias, and DVT, were extremely rare.

Discussion

Performing endovenous ablation of the GSV without division of each of the tributaries at the SFJ goes against a fundamental, long-held rule in saphenous vein surgery; however, the combined experiences with transcatheter endovenous ablation procedures have shown lower recurrence rates compared with surgical ligation and stripping. Avoiding the trauma of surgical dissection and preserving venous drainage in normal, compe-

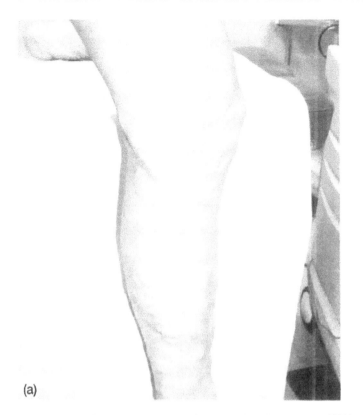
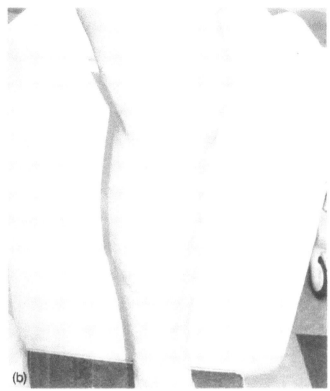

(a) Large varicose veins due to great saphenous vein (GSV) reflux are noted in the left lower extremity. (b) Significant reduction in the size of the varicose tributaries 1 month following endovenous laser ablation of the incompetent GSV. (Images courtesy of Robert Min.)

tent tributaries while removing only the abnormal refluxing segments may avoid neovascularization, which may explain these remarkable results.

The combined experience of multiple practitioners performing endovenous ablation over the past decade has revealed several important issues. Proximal portions of truncal veins appear to be the most difficult to successfully treat. Because these vein segments are exposed to the highest central venous pressures and are the least prone to venospasm, emptying the vein with Trendelenburg positioning, tumescent anesthesia, or by other means is especially important. Since transfer of thermal energy to the vein walls via direct contact with the laser fiber tip, RF electrode, or RF coil is the predominant mechanism of action of endovenous ablation, maximizing this contact will optimize the vein wall damage and eventual fibrosis. Doses of energy continue to be more precisely determined and relate to the duration of contact of a particular segment; proximal segments appear to require more prolonged exposure for successful closure.

An additional observation has been that most treatment failures seem to occur within the first year following treatment, with the majority of these becoming evident by 6 months. These failures likely represent inadequate vein wall heating with thrombus recanalization. This may be the result of too rapid laser fiber or electrode withdrawal or insufficient vein emptying, resulting in poor energy transfer to the vein wall. True recanalization of treated veins can occur, but is uncommon. Additionally, initial vein diameter is unrelated to procedural success, and there appears to be no upper size limit if adequate vein emptying is achieved. Veins with initial upright diameters in excess of 20–30 mm have been successfully closed with endovenous thermal ablation.

Many of the exclusion criteria for sclerotherapy are also relative contraindications for endovenous ablation, including dependency upon the saphenous system for venous drainage due to significant deep venous obstruction, recent DVT, non-palpable pedal pulses, inability to ambulate, general poor health, or women who are pregnant or nursing. Additional relative contraindications to all catheter-based endovenous ablation techniques are nontraversable vein segments either due to thrombosis or extreme tortuosity. Fortunately, these are uncommon findings, and should be recognized on pretreatment venous duplex ultrasound mapping.

The ease and success of varicose vein treatment has taken an enormous step forward with these new endovenous ablative procedures. Patients can now be reliably improved with a minimally invasive technique with little associated downtime or morbidity. Along with the increasing recognition of the importance of superficial vein disease in the pathophysiology of more serious disorders such as chronic venous insufficiency and venous ulceration, the incidence, along with the associated costs and disability, of these complications should be diminished substantially as endovenous thermal ablation is increasingly applied.

1. McMullin GM, Coleridge Smith PD, Scurr JH. Objective assessment of high ligation without stripping the long saphenous vein. Br J Surg 1991; 78: 1139–42.

2. Stonebridge PA, Chalmers N, Beggs I, Bradbury AW, Ruckley CV. Recurrent varicose veins: a varicographic analysis leading to a new practical classification. Br J Surg 1995; 82: 60–2.

3. Rutgers PH, Kitslaar PJEHM. Randomized trial of stripping versus high ligation combined with sclerotherapy in the treatment of incompetent greater saphenous vein. Am J Surg 1994; 168: 311–15.

4. Weiss RA, Weiss MA. Controlled radiofrequency endovenous occlusion using a unique radiofrequency catheter under duplex guidance to eliminate saphenous varicose vein reflux: a 2-year follow-up. Dermatol Surg 2002; 28: 38–42.

5. Merchant RF, DePalma RG, Kabnick LS. Endovascular obliteration of saphenous reflux: a multicenter study. J Vasc Surg 2002; 35: 1190–6.

6. Kistner RL. Endovascular obliteration of the greater saphenous vein: the Closure procedure. Jpn J Phlebol 2002; 13: 325–33.

7. Pichot O, Kabnick LS, Creton D, et al. Duplex ultrasound scan findings two years after great saphenous vein radiofrequency endovenous obliteration. J Vasc Surg 2004; 39: 189–95.

8. Nicolini P; Closure Group. Treatment of primary varicose veins by endovenous obliteration with the VNUS closure system: results of a prospective multicentre study. Eur J Vasc Endovasc Surg 2005; 29: 433–9.

9. Merchant RF, Pichot O, Myers KA. Four-year follow-up on endovascular radiofrequency obliteration of great saphenous reflux. Dermatol Surg 2005; 31: 129–34.

10. Lurie F, Creton D, Eklof B, et al. Prospective randomised study of endovenous radiofrequency obliteration (closure) versus ligation and vein stripping (EVOLVeS): two-year follow-up. Eur J Vasc Endovasc Surg 2005; 29: 67–73.

11. Merchant RF, Pichot O, for the Closure study group. Long-term outcomes of endovenous radiofrequency obliteration of saphenous reflux as a treatment for superficial venous insufficiency. J Vasc Surg 2005; 42: 502–9.

12. Merchant RF, Frisbie JS, Kistner RL. Endovenous radiofrequency obliteration of saphenous vein reflux. In: Pearce WH, Matsumura JS, Yao JS, eds. Trends in Vascular Surgery 2006. Evanston, IL: Greenwood Academic, 2007: 429–42.

13. Kianifard B, Holdstock JM, Whiteley MS. Radiofrequency ablation (VNUS closure) does not cause neo-vascularisation at the groin at one year: results of a case controlled study. Surgeon 2006; 4: 71–4.

14. Rautio T, Ohinmaa A, Perälä J, et al. Endovenous obliteration versus conventional stripping operation in the treatment of primary varicose veins: a randomized controlled trial with comparison of costs. J Vasc Surg 2002; 35: 958–65.

15. Lurie F, Creton D, Eklof B, et al. Prospective randomized study of endovenous radiofrequency obliteration (closure procedure) versus ligation and stripping in a selected patient population (EVOLVeS Study). J Vasc Surg 2003; 38: 207–14.

16. Stötter L, Schaaf I, Bockelbrink A, et al. Radiowellenobliteration, invagination or cryostripping: Which is the best tolerated treatment by the patients?] Phlebologie 2005; 34: 19–24.

17. Hinchliffe RJ, Ubhi J, Beech A, Ellison J, Braithwaite BD. A prospective randomised controlled trial of VNUS closure versus surgery for the treatment of recurrent long saphenous varicose veins. Eur J Vasc Endovasc Surg 2006; 31: 212–18.

18. Peden EK, Lumsden AB. RF ablation of incompetent perforators–description of a technique using VNUS ClosureRFS stylet. Endovasc Today 2007; Jan: S15–17.

19. Lumsden AB, Peden EK. Clinical use of the new VNUS ClosureFAST radiofrequency catheter. Endovasc Today 2007; Jan: S7–10.

20. Boné C. Tratamiento endoluminal de las varices con laser de diodo. Estudio preliminary. [Endoluminal treatment of varices with diode laser. Preliminary study.] Rev Patol Vasc 1999; V: 35–46.

21. Navarro L, Min R, Boné C. Endovenous laser: a new minimally invasive method of treatment for varicose veins – preliminary observations using an 810 nm diode laser. Dermatol Surg 2001; 27: 117–22.

22. Min R, Zimmet S, Isaacs M, Forrestal M. Endovenous laser treatment of the incompetent greater saphenous vein. J Vasc Interv Radiol 2001; 12: 1167–71.

23. Timperman PE, Sichlau M, Ryu RK. Greater energy delivery improves treatment success of endovenous laser treatment of incompetent saphenous veins. J Vasc Interv Radiol 2004; 15: 1061–3.

24. Timperman PE. Prospective evaluation of higher energy great saphenous vein endovenous laser treatment. J Vasc Interv Radiol 2005; 16: 791–4.

25. Proebstle TM, Krummenauer F, Gul D, Knop J. Nonocclusion and early reopening of the great saphenous vein after endovenous laser treatment is fluence dependent. Dermatol Surg 2004; 30: 174–8.

26. Min R, Khilnani N, Zimmet SE. Endovenous laser treatment of saphenous vein reflux: long term results. J Vasc Interv Radiol 2003; 14: 991–6.

27. Min R, Khilnani N. Endovenous laser ablation of varicose veins. J Cardiovasc Surg 2005; 46: 395–405.

28. Proebstle TM, Gul D, Lehr HA, et al. Infrequent early recanalization of great saphenous vein after endovenous laser treatment. J Vasc Surg 2003; 38: 511–16.

29. Oh CK, Jung DS, Jang HS, Kwon KS. Endovenous laser surgery of the incompetent greater saphenous vein with a 980-nm diode laser. Dermatol Surg 2003; 29: 1135–40.

30. Sadick NS, Wasser S. Combined endovascular laser with ambulatory phlebectomy for the treatment of superficial venous incompetence: a 2-year perspective. J Cosmet Laser Ther 2004; 6: 44–9.

31. Perkowski P, Ravi R, Gowda RC, et al. Endovenous laser ablation of the saphenous vein for treatment of venous insufficiency and varicose veins: early results from a large single-center experience. J Endovasc Ther 2004; 11: 132–8.

Introduction

History has witnessed various approaches to the treatment of varicose veins. The trend toward less invasive ambulatory treatments, begun in the 1950's, escalated as tumescent anesthesia and endovenous therapies emerged. However, an understanding of both the historical and current surgical approaches to treatment of venous disease is helpful in developing a comprehensive approach to phlebology.

Surgical indications

Patients present for evaluation and treatment of both cosmetic and medical venous pathology. After a thorough history, physical examination, and testing, the diagnosis and treatment options are presented to the patient. Most patients consult a physician because of symptoms related to their venous disease. Symptoms of venous disease include aching, itching, pain, fatigue, heaviness, nocturnal cramps, and swelling in the legs. These symptoms worsen as the day progresses and many women report symptoms to be maximal on the first day of the menses. Patients may elevate their legs, take prescription or over-the-counter pain medications, wear compression hose, or in other ways, alter their lifestyle in an attempt to relieve their symptoms.

Indications for surgical intervention include progressive varicose veins with symptoms altering the patient's activities of daily living, or complications of varicose veins such as superficial thrombophlebitis, bleeding from high-pressure venous blebs, or advanced skin changes of chronic venous insufficiency (ankle hyperpigmentation, eczema, subcutaneous lipodermatosclerosis, atrophie blanche, or frank ulceration). At other times, it is the appearance of asymptomatic telangiectatic blemishes or protuberant varicosities that stimulates consultation. These cosmetic findings, when associated with underlying venous reflux, may be the only indication for surgical intervention. Lastly, some patients have a family history of serious venous disease and are concerned that their condition will progress and cause significant morbidity.

Surgical objectives

Objectives of treatment for varicose veins include correction of the hydrostatic forces of axial (saphenous) reflux, and the hydrodynamic forces of perforator vein reflux, and removal of the varicose vein clusters in a cosmetic fashion.

The optimal treatment should improve venous function, and enhance cosmesis with minimal complications. The procedures are most often provided in an office-based ambulatory setting and are performed under local anesthesia, with minimal downtime for the patient.

Primary varicose vein intervention

The techniques of venous surgery are well described in standard surgical texts. Familiarity with the historical surgical options is beneficial if one is to possess comprehensive knowledge in the field of phlebology. There are times when the phlebologist may be called upon to perform one of the more traditional surgical procedures, based upon resources available to the physician or patient or the underlying pathology present in a particular individual.

High ligation of the great saphenous vein (GSV) and tributaries at the saphenofemoral junction (SFJ) or the small saphenous vein (SSV) at the saphenopopliteal junction (SPJ) was practiced to control gravitational reflux while preserving the vein for subsequent arterial bypass. The saphenous vein was largely preserved after high ligation, but reflux was not controlled in the long term. In addition, ligation of the groin tributaries contributed to neovascularization and recurrent varicose veins.

High ligation and complete stripping of the GSV and/or SSV continued after high ligation alone was abandoned. This procedure was often combined with "stab" phlebectomy, where the bulging tributary veins were removed via multiple 2- to 3-inch incisions, with individual ligation of the varicose veins. These procedures were associated with a high recurrence rate, lengthy recovery, and unsightly scarring.

Duplex ultrasound mapping is now used to accurately identify the extent of saphenous and tributary vein reflux and its variability, as well as incompetent perforating veins. With the diagnostic capabilities of duplex ultrasound, the surgical options for control of reflux evolved. Rather than performing a blind, standardized procedure, the object changed to providing precise treatment of the incompetent veins while preserving the normally functioning veins, by eliminating saphenous vein reflux, incompetent perforator veins, and refluxing tributary veins.

Thus, the trend has been away from more invasive stripping and ligation procedures and toward less invasive procedures, frequently guided by real-time ultrasound imaging. High ligation of the GSV, preserving the groin tributaries, with perforation-invagination (PIN) stripping of the refluxing portion of the GSV or SSV replaced ligation alone and the traditional stripping for axial reflux. PIN stripping utilizes a narrow gauge stripping instrument and results in invagination of the vein, thus reducing the damage caused to surrounding tissues compared with traditional stripping. Although not usually necessary in PIN stripping, tourniquet use is important if massive varices or the Klippel-Trenaunay syndrome are present. Other techniques to decrease hematomas after downward stripping include tumescent anesthesia and post-treatment compression.

The below-knee portion of the GSV is not treated unless duplex ultrasound reveals that it is refluxing, dilated, and associated with varicose tributaries. Treating only the thigh portion removes the gravitational reflux and detaches the thigh perforating veins, thus lowering the risk of injury to the saphenous nerve, which is in close proximity to the GSV in the calf. Treatment of the refluxing SSV has evolved in a similar fashion. These procedures meet the objectives of being completed under local anesthesia in an office setting with minimal scarring.

Newer techniques to remove the saphenous veins from the superficial venous circulation involve ablation using heat, generated by radiofrequency (RF) or laser sources. Like PIN stripping and phlebectomy, these procedures have the advantage of being performed under local anesthesia in an outpatient or office setting. Reports showing the safety and efficacy of RF and laser ablation of the GSV are encouraging. Five-year data are promising and confirm permanent ablation, demonstrating recurrence rates lower than those with standard surgical ligation and stripping.

Treatment of perforator veins

Incompetent perforators can be localized with duplex ultrasound and interrupted by several techniques, including the Linton procedure, open surgical ligation of the perforator, subfascial endoscopic perforator surgery (SEPS), ultrasound-guided sclerotherapy, or ultrasound-guided endovenous treatment with RF or laser. As in other areas of phlebology, trends have been toward the less invasive procedures.

The Linton procedure involved open surgical ligation of all identifiable perforators in the medial leg. The procedure required general or regional anesthesia and a long incision in the medial leg through the unhealthy skin, and was associated with high rates of infection and an extended healing process. This approach has been abandoned in favor of less invasive procedures. Simple ligation of an incompetent perforator when located in healthy skin may prove effective. This can be accomplished under local anesthesia in an ambulatory setting.

SEPS was designed to interrupt the incompetent perforator veins that contribute to the development and progression of lipodermatosclerosis in the medial leg and ankle. SEPS is performed through incisions proximal to the unhealthy skin and avoids the complications of the Linton procedure. Access to the distal leg perforators may be limited with SEPS. Some centers in Europe perform SEPS under local anesthesia with intravenous sedation, but most centers in the United States use regional or general anesthesia. SEPS requires endoscopic training and equipment, factors that have deterred its wide acceptance.

Ultrasound-guided approaches to the treatment of incompetent perforators are promising. Foam sclerotherapy and open surgical ligation of individual perforators appear to be as effective and less expensive, and obviate the need for regional or general anesthesia and the operating theater. Emerging technology is encouraging for ultrasound-guided treatment of incompetent perforators by endovenous thermal techniques using RF or laser.

Treatment of recurrent varicose veins

Persistence of the saphenous vein, neovascularization, and incompetent perforator veins are the most frequent sources of reflux contributing to recurrent varicose veins. Prior to the advent of duplex ultrasonography, saphenous vein stripping was a "blind" procedure, and the surgeon could easily miss the underlying pathology such as an accessory or duplication of the saphenous vein, leading to early recurrent reflux. Two-thirds of patients presenting for surgical relief of recurrent varicosities required treatment of a "retained" saphenous vein as part of the repeat procedure. A "retained" GSV may actually be a duplicated or accessory saphenous vein in the mid portion of the thigh. A detailed preoperative duplex scan will alert the surgeon to the presence of these venous anomalies and should substantially reduce the rate of recurrence.

Recurrent varicose veins secondary to neovascularization have also been a significant problem. In fact, neovascularization was found in 49% of cases of recurrent varicose veins after stripping, and has been linked to ligation of the groin tributaries. In this situation, late recurrence after vein stripping is often associated with a visible network of refluxing veins from the old SFJ, connecting with the varicose veins. This has challenged the old dogma that stressed the importance of ligating the pudendal and inferior epigastric vessels during ligation at the SFJ, and it is now theorized that avoiding ligation of these vessels may reduce the incidence of neovascularization. The newer thermal ablation techniques also avoid this potential complication by closing the vein below the drainage point of these vessels. The surgical control of neovascularization once it is present may prove elusive, and is best left to ultrasound-guided sclerotherapy.

Treatment of tributary varicose veins

The optimal surgical therapy for tributary (branch) varicose veins is ambulatory phlebectomy, which involves the removal of the tributaries through small incisions, using surgical hooks. This procedure is described in Chapter 13.

Compression and ambulation are the cornerstones of successful postoperative treatment of venous insufficiency. Foam padding, short stretch and/or elastic bandages, and 30–40 mmHg compression stockings all may be utilized to achieve effective compression following surgical intervention. Early ambulation and return to routine activities is strongly encouraged, in order to minimize postoperative discomfort and to avoid rare complications, such as deep vein thrombosis (DVT).

With proper preoperative evaluation and procedure selection, modern surgical procedures are all effective methods of reducing or eliminating the symptoms and sequelae of chronic venous insufficiency. These procedures meet the objectives of being minimally invasive, ambulatory, and cosmetically appealing.

Each procedure has its own risks, which generally include pain, ecchymosis, paresthesia, nerve dysfunction, hyperpigmentation, scarring, hematoma, superficial thrombophlebitis, lymphocele, lymphedema, neovascularization, infection, and DVT. With proper preoperative evaluation, postoperative compression, and early ambulation, the incidence of all of these complications has been reduced and patient acceptance of these procedures is significantly improved.

Surgical recommendations for treatment of varicose veins are based upon years of experience. A greater understanding of the etiologies of primary and recurrent varicose veins and the opportunity for pre- or intraoperative ultrasound imaging have led to less invasive and more precise procedures. The future promises even better results as we critically observe the results of our treatments.

1. Weiss RA, Feied CF, Weiss MA, eds. Vein Diagnosis and Treatment – A Comprehensive approach. New York: McGraw-Hill, 2001.

2. Bergan JJ. Surgical management of primary and recurrent varicose veins. In: Gloviczki P, Yao JST, eds. Handbook of Venous Disorders, 2nd edn. New York: Arnold, 2001: 287–302.

3. McMullin GM, Coleridge Smith PD, Scurr JH. Objective assessment of high ligation without stripping the long saphenous vein. Br J Surg 1991; 78: 1139–42.

4. Durkin MT, Turton EP, Scott DJ, Berridge DC. A prospective randomised trial of PIN versus conventional stripping in varicose vein surgery. Ann R Coll Surg Engl 1999; 81: 171–4.

5. Chandler JG, Pichot O, Sessa C, et al. Treatment of primary venous insufficiency by endovenous saphenous vein obliteration. Vasc Surg 2000; 34: 201–14.

6. Min RJ, Zimmet SE, Isaacs MN, Forrestal MD. Endovenous laser treatment of the incompetent greater saphenous vein. J Vasc Interv Radiol 2001; 12: 1167–71

7. Dunn CW, Kabnick LS, Merchant RF, et al. Endovascular radiofrequency obliteration using 90°C for treatment of great saphenous vein. Ann Vasc Surg 2006; 20: 625–9.

8. Gibson KD, Ferris BL, Polissar N, Neradliek B, Pepper D. Endovenous laser treatment of the short saphenous vein: efficacy and complications. J Vasc Surg 2007; 45: 795–803.

9. Papadakis K, Christodoulou C, Christopoulos D, et al. Number and anatomical distribution of incompetent thigh perforating veins. Br J Surg 1989; 76: 581–84.

10. Gloviczki P. Subfascial endoscopic perforator surgery: indications and results. Vasc Med 1999; 4: 173–80.

11. Bergan JJ. Varicose veins: hooks, clamps and suction. Application of new techniques to enhance varicose vein surgery. Semin Vasc Surg 2002; 15: 21–6.

12. Cabrera J, Cabrera Jr A, Garcia-Olmedo A. Treatment of varicose long saphenous veins with sclerosant in microfoam form: long-term outcomes. Phlebology 2000; 15: 19–23.

13. Jones L, Braithwaite BD, Selwyn D, et al. Neovascularization is the principal cause of varicose vein recurrence: results of a randomized trial of stripping the long saphenous vein. Eur J Vasc Endovasc Surg 1996; 12: 442–5.

14. Kostas T, Ioannou CV, Touloupakis E, et al. Recurrent varicose veins after surgery: a new appraisal of a common and complex problem in vascular surgery. Eur J Endovasc Surg 2004; 27: 275–82.

15. Lurie F, Creton D, Eklof B, et al. Prospective randomized study of endovenous radiofrequency obliteration (Closure procedure versus ligation and stripping in a selected patient population (EVOLVeS study). J Vasc Surg 2003; 38: 207–14.

16. Henriet JP. Three years' experience with polidocanol foam in treatment of reticular varices and varicosities. Phlebologie 1999; 52: 277–82.

Definition

Ambulatory phlebectomy is a technique that was initially described thousands of years ago and was reintroduced in the 1950's by a Swiss dermatologist, Dr Robert Muller. Muller described the removal of segments of varicose veins, under local anesthesia, on an outpatient basis. Excluding telangiectasias and the proximal few centimeters of the great or small saphenous vein, varicosities of any size and from any location are accessible and can be removed with ambulatory phlebectomy.

Ambulatory phlebectomy, alone or in combination with ablative procedures or stripping applied to the saphenous veins, is frequently performed in many medical facilities throughout the world. Although most commonly used to remove varicosities of the legs, it is also effective in the treatment of varicose veins of the feet, hands, and face, areas that are often avoided. Refinements to this minimally invasive technique have made it possible for even elderly patients to undergo treatment of varicose veins.

Indications for ambulatory phlebectomy

Ambulatory phlebectomy is an elective procedure, so there are no emergency indications. Asymptomatic patients may present for treatment of spider or varicose veins on the legs, hands, or face because of their cosmetic appearance, fear of progression of their venous disease, a strong family history of varicose veins, or fear of future complications of venous disease. The initial evaluation will identify those patients with associated venous reflux and the vessels that require treatment. Symptomatic patients often have saphenous insufficiency, but even tributary varicose veins with reflux can result in symptoms. While conservative therapy — including graduated compression stockings, elevation, exercise, and weight control — may be recommended, it is recognized as a temporizing measure that many patients do not or cannot pursue indefinitely. Rather, they seek definitive treatment, which may include removal of these varicose veins by ambulatory phlebectomy.

Other patients present for ambulatory phlebectomy because of complications of their varicose veins. These complications may include recurrent superficial thrombophlebitis, bleeding, skin changes of chronic venous insufficiency, chronic painful edema, corona phlebectasia, hyperpigmentation, dermatitis, and healed or active venous ulcers.

Contraindications to ambulatory phlebectomy

Patients with infection, dermatitis, or cellulitis of the area to be treated should have the infectious process controlled prior to the phlebectomy. Severe peripheral edema or lymphedema should also be controlled, since edema results in an increased risk of infection following any varicose vein procedure. Also, the surgeon should verify deep system competency prior to extensive phlebectomy.

Patients who are seriously ill, non-ambulatory, or have significant arterial stenosis are best treated with conservative care. In patients with severe cardiovascular disease, pulmonary disease, uncontrolled diabetes, clotting disorders, or problems with immunity, the medical condition must be stabilized prior to intervention, and medical clearance must be sought from their primary physician in these cases. Ambulatory phlebectomy is delayed in pregnant patients to allow at least 12 weeks post-partum recovery for the varicosities to spontaneously regress prior to intervention.

Reports of medication allergies are not uncommon and warrant investigation, although they do not necessarily constitute a contraindication to ambulatory phlebectomy. Possible reactions include a vasovagal response, histamine responses ranging from urticaria to anaphylactic reactions, and an excitation response due to epinephrine containing anesthetics. Iodine allergy may prompt the use of an alternative prepping solution. A local anesthetic "allergy" may be related to the anesthetic itself, a side-effect of the preservative in multidose bottles, or the epinephrine in the local anesthetic (tremor or palpitations). Allergy testing may help to identify the truly allergic patient. Reactions may be avoided by changing the anesthetic or eliminating the epinephrine. Facilities should have a plan for dealing with the unlikely event of an allergic reaction.

Technique of ambulatory phlebectomy

Preoperative evaluation and marking

Patients are interviewed and examined to determine if their complaint is cosmetic or if it is a medical vein condition with underlying axial or perforator vein reflux. Transillumination devices may be utilized for identifying varicose tributaries, reticular varicose veins, and veins that feed the telangiectasias. Testing for reflux includes at a minimum a handheld Doppler examination, but preferably duplex ultrasound should be used in all patients. This evaluation forms the framework for treatment recommendations.

Preoperative marking is critical to success and can initially be done while the patient is standing, using surgical pens or permanent markers. However, final marking of the varicose veins in the supine position allows more precise localization and marking of the varicose segments. Transillumination or ultrasound imaging may be used to more accurately detect and mark the varicose veins. If the patient has been wearing compression before the procedure, standing for 20 minutes without compression hose may allow better visualization of the varicosities. If more than one procedure is planned in a particular extremity, a detailed plan for removal of all the varicosities should be made before the initial procedure.

Surgical plan

If the saphenofemoral junction and great saphenous vein and/or the saphenopopliteal junction and small saphenous vein are proven to be incompetent by duplex examination, treatment of the truncal reflux should be performed before or in conjunction with the ambulatory phlebectomy. In cases of extremities with very large varicosities, the more heavily involved areas should be treated first. It is best to start at the distal portion of the leg.

Staging the procedures is particularly beneficial in elderly patients or patients with extensive varicosities, since it allows for a shorter procedure, a lower dose of local anesthetic, and immediate discharge, with less discomfort and earlier ambulation. The interval between phlebectomy sessions is usually no longer than 1–2 weeks. Staged phlebectomy of varicosities in the same extremity may result in acute superficial thrombophlebitis in the area of retained varicose veins. This may delay or make the second procedure more difficult.

Local anesthesia

The introduction of tumescent local anesthesia by Dr Jeff Klein allowed phlebological surgery to move into the office setting. The tumescent local anesthetic is diluted, to allow the use of larger volumes in order to treat a wider area. Lidocaine concentrations as low as 0.1% can be quite effective, with less risk of reaching levels of toxicity, even when using up to 35 mg/kg. The typical Klein solution includes normal (0.9%) saline (1000 cm³), lidocaine 1% with epinephrine (100 cm³), and 8.4% sodium bicarbonate (10 cm³). In patients who are over 60 years of age, it may be advisable to use lidocaine without epinephrine. If the amount of local anesthesia to be used is more than the recommended maximum dose, the procedure must be staged into two or more sessions, which should be no longer than 1–2 weeks apart, as noted above.

Infiltration of the local anesthetic is done immediately prior to the procedure. Standard syringes, pressure bags, or a mechanical pump may be utilized to assist with the administration of the tumescent local anesthesia. A ⅜-inch 30-gauge needle is used to raise a skin wheal, and a 1½-inch 25-gauge needle is used to infiltrate the subcutaneous tissue. A spinal needle may also be used to anesthetize the subcutaneous perivenous tissue, and is also used around the saphenous veins in the venous fascial compartment under ultrasound guidance. Infiltration is begun distally and progresses proximally, all the way to the groin if necessary.

Klein describes the use of a tumescent infusion cannula with multiple side-ports and a blunt tip requiring a small skin incision for insertion. The benefits of this technique include less patient discomfort and rapid delivery of the tumescent anesthesia solution.

Ambulatory phlebectomy technique (Figure 12.1)

Incision size and vein retrieval distinguish ambulatory phlebectomy from the older stab phlebectomy technique. The micro-incision for ambulatory phlebectomy ranges from 1 to 3 mm and is adjusted according to the size of the vein to be removed. The longer the incision, the more visible the scar will be and the greater the chance of pigmentation. An exception to this rule is when a very large vein is removed through an incision that is too small, causing stretching of the incision and making it more noticeable.

A variety of blades may be used to create the micro-incision. They vary from the classic #11 blade to 18-gauge needles, lancets, ophthalmology blades, or custom blades cut to size. Most surgeons utilize a #11 blade, which can be grasped transversely with a 4-inch needle holder. The size of the incision can be adjusted by moving the holder up and down the #11 blade.

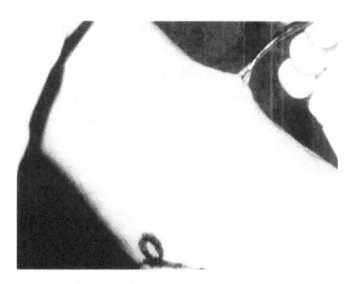

With ambulatory phlebectomy, the vein is removed in segments through small incisions or punctures. (Image courtesy of Mitchel P Goldman MD.)

The orientation of the incision is important. Vertical incisions usually leave a better cosmetic result. However, around the knee and ankle, a horizontal incision following the Langer lines is better.

The interval (distance) between the incisions varies between 1 and 5 cm according to the patient, the size and type of vein that is being removed, and the skin type. Micro-incisions may be left alone or suture strips may be placed. When the incision is longer than 4 mm, a single 6-0 nylon suture is applied to obtain a more aesthetic scar.

Various hooks have been designed for ambulatory phlebectomy.[13–15] The Muller, Oesch, Ramelet, Varady, Trauchessec, Dortu-Martimbeau, Tretbar, and Vergereau hooks are the most widely used. They differ in their sharpness and the shape of the tip and handle. Every physician performing ambulatory phlebectomy should experiment with the hooks available and then decide which one is best suited for his or her style.

The phlebectomy hook is introduced through the incision and rotated and moved in a plane perpendicular to the vein to be removed. When the vein is hooked, it is brought gently through the incision and grasped with a mosquito clamp. The clamp is never introduced into the incision. With a rotating motion, the vein is loosened and slowly avulsed. Massaging the skin with the tips of the index finger and thumb of the free hand facilitates the removal of a longer segment of vein.

Traction is continued with the mosquito clamp as the vein is removed. The vein may be divided between mosquito clamps. The clamp is rotated, rolling the vein around it as it is avulsed, freeing the vein from the surrounding connective tissue. Traction also outlines the course of the vein.

The conventional technique recommends that the tip of the mosquito clamp should be pointed upward while traction is applied. It may be useful to push the clamp with the attached vein away from the patient's leg with its tip pointed downward, applying a steady, but firm, tug on the vein. This maneuver can be steadied and made more effective by the operator resting his or her wrist and hand on the patient's leg while pushing the clamp away from the leg, regrasping and repositioning the clamp as more vein is removed.

The surgeon should always try to remove the entire segment of the vein that has been marked. Retained segments of varicosities will result in localized thrombophlebitis that will leave tender, "lumpy" areas with a tendency to leave dark pigmentation of the overlying skin.

Care should be paid to areas such as the ankle and foot, where "hooking" should be gentle and slow. The foot should be dorsiflexed to decrease the tension of the anatomic structures, including the veins. Once the vein has been hooked, it should come out easily; if it is difficult or requires a lot of traction, it is possible that the hooked structure is not the vein. The hook should be removed, then re-introduced, and another attempt should be made. Ambitious "hooking" in the ankle and foot should be avoided in order to eliminate complications such as swelling, hematomas, and nerve damage. Phlebectomy in the pretibial area should also be performed very carefully, because many lymphatic vessels are located in this area. Especially gentle technique should be used when performing

phlebectomies in the popliteal area due to the proximity of the peroneal nerve and because the skin of the back of the knee is very soft and micro-incisions are very easily enlarged by ambitious and energetic "hooking".[8,16,17]

TRIVEX phlebectomy

Transilluminated powered phlebectomy (TriVex) is another method that removes large, superficial varicose veins. Spitz developed and patented this procedure and has documented excellent results. TriVex reduces operative time, permits visualization of the varicose vein removal and can be accomplished via several 2–3 mm incisions. The TriVex procedure requires intravenous sedation/regional or general anesthesia along with tumescent local anesthesia, which limits its usefulness as an office-based procedure.[18]

Postoperative wrapping

After the procedure has been completed and bleeding has been controlled, the leg should be washed with hydrogen peroxide or sterile saline. Many dressing protocols have been used successfully by different phlebologists, but all must approximate the micro-incisions, control the serous tumescent drainage, and provide adequate graduated post-procedure compression.

Steri-strips or tape should be applied carefully to avoid tension on the skin edges. Skin irritation due to the adhesive present on the tape and blister formation from tension from inelastic strips is especially common near the knee. If there is a need for further approximation, it is best to apply a single 6-0 nylon suture to be removed in 5–7 days.

A simple hydrophilic pad or several layers of gauze are applied for absorption of tumescent drainage at the incision sites. Next, a layer of adhesive or short-stretch bandage is used in order to secure these dressings. The bandage is extremely important in order to minimize the ecchymosis and allow the patient to be discharged ambulatory. Alternatively, a class II, 30–40 mmHg graduated compression stocking is placed on top of the hydrophilic pad or absorptive material in order to apply extra pressure and keep the wrapping in place. In the elderly, this stocking can be removed at night. The bandages are removed after 1–7 days, depending on the size and location of the veins that have been removed. The compression stocking is worn for at least 2–4 weeks, depending on the amount of ecchymosis present.[2,5,11]

Discharge recommendations

All patients are asked to walk in or around the office for 10–15 minutes to check for postoperative bleeding and to be sure that the wrapping is comfortable and tolerable. They are then discharged home, and, after the first day, encouraged to walk as much as possible. It is recommended that everyone bring a driver.[1,2,11] Ice may be applied to the treated area twice a day for 10–15 minutes after the tumescent anesthesia effect has resolved (4–6 hours after completion of the procedure).

Pain control is usually accomplished with anti-inflammatory

medication, often started prior to the procedure, and continued for 5–10 days postoperatively. Acetaminophen may be added if necessary. Narcotics are infrequently needed to control post-operative pain.

The patient removes the dressings 2–3 days following surgery, or may return to the office as long as 7 days later for bandage removal and wound checks. After the wrappings are completely removed, it is recommended that the patient wear a compression stocking for 2–4 weeks and be rechecked in 1 month and then in 3 months. Once the patient is ready to be discharged, a final picture is taken of the treated area.

Ambulatory phlebectomy adequately and satisfactorily removes varicosities of different sizes, and results in a series of very acceptable microscars that are pleasing to the patient and the surgeon. Complications associated with ambulatory phlebectomy are mostly benign and resolve spontaneously.[19–21] These include hyper- or hypopigmentation, visible scars, local infection, and dressing/compression-related skin reactions. Other rare cutaneous complications include tattooing, silica granulomas, and Köbner's phenomenon.

Vascular ri   include post-procedure bleeding, hematomas, telangiectatic matting, lymphorrhea and pseudocyst, edema (foot), superficial phlebitis, and deep vein thrombosis (DVT). Neurological risks include transient or definitive numbness, and neuromas. Other general risks include vasovagal reactions and allergic reactions.[22–24]

The physician should be aware of potential risks and have standard office protocols in place for dealing with these if they occur.

1. Muller R, Joubert B. La Phlébectomie Ambulatoire: de l'Anatomie au Geste. L'Hay-Les-Roses, Switzerland: Les éditions médicales Innothéra, 1992: 105–12.
2. Ricci S, Georgiev M. Office varicose vein surgery under local anesthesia. J Dermatol Surg Oncol 1992; 18: 55–8.
3. Olivencia JA. New trends in varicose vein treatment. Iowa Med 1996; 86: 203-4
4. Olivencia JA. Varicose veins: not just a cosmetic problem. Patient Care 1996; 30: 140–58.
5. Garde C. Ambulatory phlebectomy. Dermatol Surg 1995; 21: 628–30.
6. Olivencia JA. Ambulatory phlebectomy of the foot: review of 75 cases. Dermatol Surg 1997; 23: 279-80.
7. Neuman HAM. Ambulant minisurgical phlebectomy (Editorial). J Dermatol Surg Oncol 1992; 18: 53–4.
8. Weis RA, Ramelet AA. Removal of blue periocular lower eyelid veins by ambulatory phlebectomy. Dermatol Surg 2002; 28: 43–5.
9. Olivencia JA. Ambulatory phlebectomy in the elderly: review of 100 consecutive cases. Phlebology 1997; 12: 78–80.
10. Oesch A. [Indications for and results of ambulatory varices therapy.] Ther Umsch 1991; 48: 692–6.
11. Georgiev M, Ricci S. Stab avulsion of the lesser saphenous vein. J Dermatol Surg Oncol 1993; 19: 456–64.
12. Klein JA. Tumescent technique for regional anesthesia permits lidocaine doses of 35 mg/kg for liposuction. J Dermatol Surg Oncol 1990; 16: 248–63.
13. Ramelet AA. Muller phlebectomy. A new phlebectomy hook. J Dermatol Surg Oncol 1991; 17: 814–16.
14. Van Cleef JF. [Instruments for ambulatory phlebectomy.] Phlebologie 1991; 44: 683–6.
15. Varady Z. \   chirurgische Phlebextraktion nach varady in der varizenchirurgie. Intern Diskussionsblatt 1988; 1: 8–9.
16. Fratila A, Rabe E, Kreysel H. Percutaneous minisurgical phlebectomy. Semin Dermatol 1993; 12: 117–22.
17. Olivencia JA. Maneuver to facilitate ambulatory phlebectomy. Dermatol Surg 1996; 22: 654–5.
18. Chetter IC, Mylankal KJ, Hughes H, Firtridge R. Randomized clinical trial comparing multiple stab incision phlebectomy and transilluminated powered phlebectomy for varicose veins. Br J Surg 2006; 93: 169–74.
19. Ramelet AA. Complications of ambulatory phlebectomy. Dermatol Surg 1997; 23: 947–54.
20. Goutier Y, Dortu J, Raymond-Martimbeau P. Adverse incidence and complications. In: Ambulatory Phlebectomy. Houston: PRM Editions, 1993: 111.
21. Olivencia JA. Complications of ambulatory phlebectomy: review of 1000 consecutive cases. Dermatol Surg 1997; 23: 51–4.
22. Ramelet AA. An unusual complication of ambulatory phlebectomy. Talc granuloma. Phlebologie 1991; 44: 865–71.
23. Roos de KP, Neumann, HAM. Traumatic neuroma: a rare complication following Muller's phlebectomy. J Dermatol Surg Oncol 1994; 20: 681–2.
24. Olivencia JA. Ambulatory phlebectomy: rare complication of local anesthesia: a case report and literature review. Dermatol Surg 1996; 22: 53–5.

Most patients needing varicose vein surgery or the increasingly popular endovascular thermal ablation techniques are candidates for an office procedure. Advantages of the office setting include a reduction in the risk of nosocomial infections and the comfort that the patient derives from their familiarity with the staff and the office environment. This situation has led to a renewed interest in the use of regional anesthesia, which further enhances the patient's acceptance of varicose vein treatments. Every practitioner should know the anesthetic requirements of the intended procedure. Knowledge of local anesthetic drugs — their administration, uptake, distribution, and elimination — is essential for understanding maximum dosages and toxic/allergic reactions. Premedication, patient monitoring, and essential emergency supplies are also necessary to assist practitioners in offering these cosmetically acceptable, cost-effective procedures to their patients in a safe manner. It is of utmost importance that each physician be aware of their own limitations and strive to add this knowledge to their phlebological expertise.

Anesthesia

Anesthesia is divided into two categories: general and regional (also referred to as local anesthesia). Under general anesthesia (GA), there is a total loss of body sensations and loss of consciousness. GA requires a certified registered nurse anesthetist (CRNA) or anesthesiologist.

With regional (local) anesthesia, only a region of the body is anesthetized, and the patient is either awake or mildly sedated (but always responsive). Types of local anesthesia include topical anesthesia, local infiltration (including the tumescent technique), regional field blocks, and nerve blocks (both central and peripheral). The central nerve blocks (spinal, epidural, and caudal) should only be performed by those who have had experience or advanced training to manage potential complications. The peripheral nerve blocks of the lower extremity also affect motor and sympathetic function, which are disadvantageous to early ambulant office surgery.

Infiltrative local anesthesia may be administered by most practitioners with a wide margin of safety. Regional field blocks and local infiltration are the best choices for the phlebologist administering anesthesia in the office. Regional field blocks refer to the creation of a wall of anesthesia around an operative field, leaving the site unaffected and not distorted.

The circumferential injection pattern surrounding the procedure area should block both deep and superficial nerves supplying it. Local infiltration is the direct infiltration of a wound, lesion, or operative field. The anesthetic solution bathes the nerves and nerve endings that supply the area, causing direct inhibition of neural activity. When the solution is injected intradermally, the effects are immediate but the pain of infiltration is more intense. If injected subcutaneously, the effects are delayed but the pain is lessened. The main disadvantage of local infiltrative anesthesia is the distortion of the operative site, which is due to the volume of anesthetic solution injected.

Tumescent local anesthesia

The tumescent technique of infiltrative anesthesia involves the administration of a larger volume of a more dilute anesthetic solution. It has been shown that more local anesthetic can be used over a larger area with less risk of toxicity with these dilute, epinephrine-containing solutions. Tumescent anesthesia has become widely recognized for its safety and ability to produce excellent anesthesia of the subcutaneous tissue, skin, and underlying muscle. The increased distortion (swelling) and tissue tension create a favorable operative environment for surface hook phlebectomies. The large volume is advantageous during endovenous thermal ablation procedures, as it decreases vein diameter and produces a fluid layer that insulates the surrounding tissue from the heat generated during these techniques. Perivascular ultrasound-guided tumescent infiltration of the saphenous trunks has become the anesthetic technique of choice for endovenous thermal ablation procedures.

The commercially available solution of 1% lidocaine with epinephrine 1:100 000 contains 1 g of lidocaine and 1 mg of epinephrine per 100 mL. In contrast, a tumescent local anesthetic solution may contain the same amount but diluted in 500–1000 mL of solution. Thus, the same amount of local anesthetic can be spread over a much larger area while still producing widespread, profound surgical anesthesia with decreased risk of local anesthetic toxicity.

Local anesthetics

The sensation of pain depends on the nervous system's ability to transmit information. Local anesthetics (LAs) halt the neural traffic along nerves in a predictable and reversible manner. They are available in solution, gel, ointment, and cream preparations. The strengths of LAs are denoted in percentages, which indicate the number of grams of drug per 100 units of measure (milliliters or grams). For solutions, it is important to know how many milligrams are in each milliliter in order to calculate the total dose of drug injected. Thus, a 1.5% solution contains 1.5 g of drug per 100 mL, or, in other words, 1500 mg per 100 mL or 15 mg/mL. This can be calculated by simply moving the decimal point 1 space to the right. For example, 1 mL of a 1.5% solution contains 15 mg of the drug, and 1 mL of a 0.5% solution contains 5 mg of the drug.

Local anesthetics consist of lipophilic (benzene ring) and hydrophilic (tertiary amine) portions, separated by a hydrocarbon connecting chain. Linkage of the hydrocarbon chain to the lipophilic portion is by an ester (—CO.O—) or amide (—CO.NH—) bond. The nature of this bond is the basis for classifying LAs as esters or amides. This is important because the ester local anesthetics cocaine, procaine (Novocain®), chloroprocaine (Nesacaine®), and tetracaine (Pontocaine®) are hydrolyzed in the plasma by esterases. Hydrolysis is rapid, and by-products are excreted in the urine. However, this can be a problem for patients with pseudocholinesterase deficiency and could lead to delayed systemic toxicity. A major metabolite of ester hydrolysis is p-aminobenzoic acid (PABA). This known allergen is probably the reason that the ester anesthetics have a higher incidence of allergy as compared with their amide counterparts.

The amide LAs (Table 13.1) are hydrolyzed in the liver and should be used with caution in patients with impaired liver/renal function. The amides are more widely used, due to the fact that they cause fewer allergic reactions and do not demonstrate cross-sensitivity within their group.

The most commonly used amide anesthetics

Lidocaine (Xylocaine®)
Mepivacaine (Polocaine®, Carbocaine®)
Bupivacaine (Sensorcaine®, Marcaine®)
Etidocaine (Duranest®)
Ropivacaine (Naropin®)

All LAs have the same mode of action. In low concentrations they delay and with higher concentrations completely prevent the migration of ions across the nerve membrane. This prevents the transmission of an action potential. This membrane "stabilizing" effect is seen in all excitable tissues and is also responsible for the systemic toxicity of LAs.

LAs are bacteriostatic at low concentrations and bactericidal at high concentrations. The addition of sodium bicarbonate appears to enhance this antimicrobial activity.

Different nerve fibers are blocked in a known order with increasing concentrations of LAs. The sensory nerves are blocked after the sympathetics but before the motor nerves. Therefore, it is possible to have vasodilatation (orthostatic hypotension) in an ambulating patient with a painful post-surgical leg, especially if a nerve block was performed and the sympathetics have not recovered.

The sensory nerves are blocked and return to function in a precise order. The sensation of pain is carried by small unmyelinated "C" nerve fibers. These are blocked first but return to function last (Table 13.2). Therefore, patients will be able to feel other sensations such as temperature, touch, pressure, and stretch while still being insensitive to pain.

The "selective blocking action" of local anesthetics on sensory nerves

Onset		Return
1st	Pain	3rd
2nd	Temperature	2nd
3rd	Touch	1st

Commercially prepared single-dose vials of LAs contain hydrochloride salt solutions, which are acidified to pH 6.5 to favor the water-soluble ionized form. These single-dose solutions are usually marked MPF (methylparaben-free). Multiple-dose vials contain an antimicrobial preservative (methylparaben, 1 mg/mL). Methylparaben can be a potent allergen, and its potential cytotoxicity precludes its use in spinal, epidural, and intravenous regional anesthesia.

When epinephrine is added to LAs, the solutions must be made even more acidic (pH 3.3–5.5) to prevent oxidation of the catecholamine. An antioxidant, sodium metabisulfite 0.5 mg/mL, is added to retard breakdown, and citric acid 0.2 mg/mL is also added as a stabilizer. Using preservative-free LAs from single-dose vials and adding epinephrine at the time of use can avoid both the additives and excessive acidity. The addition of epinephrine prolongs the duration of analgesia by constricting blood vessels and slowing absorption, thus minimizing toxicity and leaving a relatively bloodless field. However, its use is contraindicated in the fingers, toes, and penis. Epinephrine may induce adverse effects (Table 13.3) and should be used cautiously in patients with heart disease or on beta-blockers. The optimal concentration of epinephrine is 1:200 000. Tissue necrosis has been reported with concentrations greater than 1:100 000. Neuritis, paralysis, and slough have been observed following the injection of lidocaine–epinephrine solutions with a concentration of 1.5% or greater.

Adverse effects of epinephrine

Central nervous system
Nervousness
Tremors
Headaches

Cardiovascular system
Palpitations
Tachycardia
Hypertension
Chest pain

Mepivacaine seems to have intrinsic vasoconstrictor action and can be used without the addition of epinephrine. The addition of epinephrine does not significantly prolong anesthesia with Mepivacaine. Ropivacaine also appears to produce vasoconstriction and has a longer duration of action than mepivacaine or lidocaine with epinephrine.

Allergy to amide LAs is very rare. Taking a good history is extremely important. The described reactions are usually related to the addition of epinephrine (palpitations, increased blood pressure) or to their mechanism of action (lightheadedness). Many more allergies have been reported to the methylparaben and sodium metabisulfite additives than to pure amide LAs. Preservative-free solutions should be used in known hypersensitive individuals.

Lidocaine is the most widely used LA in the United States. It has a rapid onset of action but a short duration of anesthesia, and usually requires the addition of epinephrine. Mepivacaine also has a rapid onset of action, but has a longer duration of action than lidocaine, making epinephrine addition unnecessary. In adults, it is less toxic than lidocaine and causes less vasodilatation. Mepivacaine is more widely used in Europe. Bupivacaine has a long duration of anesthesia but a slow onset, whereas ropivacaine has a rapid onset with a long duration, similar to bupivacaine.

Dosage

The maximum recommended doses of local anesthetics found on drug package inserts and in reference books are at best "estimates" (Table 12.6). There are so many factors that affect absorption, distribution, and metabolism of these drugs that the best guidelines have come from clinical practice. However, if placed where not intended (i.e., a larger blood vessel), these safe doses may become gross overdoses and may lead to unwanted systemic reactions. Therefore, it is imperative that all members of the operative team be well versed in the signs of local anesthetic toxicity.

For normal healthy adults, the maximum recommended dose of lidocaine with epinephrine is 7 mg/kg of body weight (not to exceed 500 mg) according to the manufacturer. Dr Jeffery Klein's studies show that 35 mg/kg is safe when using a tumescent technique with dilute lidocaine and epinephrine

for vein surgery of the lower extremities. Epinephrine-induced vasoconstriction is rapid enough to prevent rapid absorption of the dilute lidocaine, even with rapid rates of delivery. Klein's formula is 1 g of lidocaine, 1 mg of epinephrine, and 10 mmol of sodium bicarbonate per liter of normal saline or lactated Ringer's (LR) solution. It is a misconception that LR is buffered and thus does not require neutralization with bicarbonate. LR just contains lactate, which is converted to bicarbonate only after systemic absorption and is metabolized by the liver.

Administration

The infiltration of the anesthetic solution can be a painful experience for the patient. Premedication is helpful as is the anxious patient, as is the reassuring demeanor of the operative team. Conscious sedation may be used for the use of anesthetic infiltration, but, once this has been completed, it is no longer necessary. Distracting the patient with conversation ("vocal anesthesia") and informing them what they should expect also help to allay anxiety.

To minimize the pain from the needle punctures, slightly squeezing or stretching the skin with the finger and thumb of the hand not holding the syringe may decrease the perception of pain. Small anesthetic wheels made with 30-gauge needles can be connected by larger, longer needles, requiring fewer punctures. One should always inject from a previously anesthetized area toward one that is not.

Tissue irritation and pain with local anesthetics is due to many factors. Most anesthetic solutions are acidic (pH 6.5), especially those containing epinephrine (pH 2). Neutralizing epinephrine-containing solutions to a more physiologic pH by adding 1 mL of NaCl sodium bicarbonate for every 10 mL of anesthetic may reduce the pain of injection. Alternatively, plain solutions can be mixed with epinephrine (1:1000) and the pH of the original solution (pH 5.5) retained, or plain and epinephrine-containing solutions can be mixed to lower the acid levels. Slow injection allows more time for the stretch receptors to become accustomed to the volume being injected. This may explain why intradermal injections are more painful than subcutaneous injections. Warming of the solutions that have been created with decreased pain.

Technique

Technique improves with experience. Appropriate equipment is important for the safe and effective delivery of local anesthetics. Gloves and protective eyewear should be worn when there may be contact with blood and other body fluids. The area should be cleansed with alcohol or another disinfectant prior to injection. The anesthetic solution need not injected under sterile conditions.

Smaller needles are less painful but harder to inject through. Longer needles will cover a larger area with a single puncture. A 30- to 32-gauge ½-inch needle is used to make small subcutaneous wheals. The wheals can also be connected with a 25- or 23-gauge 1- to 2-inch needle. There are 22-gauge

Table 12.6 Manufacturers' suggested dose limits for each local anesthetic

Drug	Suggested maximum
Lidocaine	300 mg
	500 mg + epinephrine 5 µg/mL (1:200 000)
Mepivacaine	400 mg
	500 mg + epinephrine
Bupivacaine	175 mg
	225 mg + epinephrine 5 µg/mL (1:200 000)
Ropivacaine	200 mg*

*Commercial preparation with epinephrine not sold in US.

4-inch needles with a cutting bevel that penetrate the skin more easily than commonly used spinal needles. Many different blunt, reusable, variable length and diameter needles are available for high-volume infiltration.

Syringes should have a Luer-Lok tip to avoid separation from the needle during injection. Syringes of 10, 20, and 30 cm³ work well. Larger syringes are hard to inject with unless the needle has a large bore, and an overuse injury of the thumb may develop over time. For a practice with a moderate volume of large surgical cases, an infusion device is well worth the price. This can be as simple as a pressure bag with high-pressure tubing connected to a control handle or a peristaltic infusion pump with dual foot controls and an adjustable infusion rate.

Most LAs do not cause significant tissue reaction except when epinephrine is added. Most local reactions are due to the injection process, and include pain, ecchymosis, hematoma (especially in anticoagulated patients), infection (poor sterile technique), and nerve damage secondary to needle laceration or neurotoxicity.

Toxicity

Systemic reactions may occur with both high and low blood levels of local anesthetics. Allergic, anaphylactic, and idiosyncratic responses may be seen with low blood levels, while central nervous system (CNS) and cardiovascular toxicity occur with high blood levels. Any circumstance that creates increased absorption or impaired metabolism will lead to higher blood levels and potential systemic toxicity. Fortunately, the cerebral effects (respiratory arrest) of LAs precede the cardiac effects (cardiac arrest), except for bupivacaine. For this reason, ropivacaine may be a better choice when a long-acting anesthetic is needed.

The cerebral effects of all local anesthetics are described in Table 13.5. The inhibitory centers of the CNS are more sensitive to local anesthetics, so there will always be excitement prior to depression of the CNS. If levels rise too fast, these signs of anesthetic toxicity may not be appreciated and the patient may lose consciousness and begin to convulse.

As already mentioned, ester anesthetics (cocaine, procaine, chloroprocaine, and tetracaine) are hydrolyzed in the plasma by cholinesterase produced in the liver. Their use can be a problem for patients with pseudocholinesterase deficiency (1 in 2500).

Drugs that inhibit the hepatic enzyme cytochrome P450 3A4 (CYP3A4) interfere with the metabolism of amide local anesthetics, slowing the rate at which they are eliminated from the body. Common drugs that may increase the toxicity of lidocaine and other amide local anesthetics can be found in Table 13.6. For further information regarding lidocaine drug interactions, see http://www.liposuction.com/pharmacology/drug_interact.php.

Common drugs known to interact with lidocaine

Class of drugs	Drug	Trade name
Antibiotics	Ciprofloxacin	Cipro
	Clarithromycin	Biaxin
	Erythromycin	
Antidepressants	Amitriptyline	Elavil
	Fluoxetine	Prozac
	Paroxetine	Paxil
	Sertraline	Zoloft
Antifungals	Fluconazole	Diflucan
	Itraconazole	Sporanox
	Ketoconazole	Nizoral
	Miconazole	Monistat
Antihistamines (H₂ blockers)	Cimetidine	Tagamet
Antiseizure medications	Divalproex	Depakote
	Phenytoin	Dilantin
Benzodiazepines	Alprazolam	Xanax
	Diazepam	Valium
	Flurazepam	Dalmane
	Midazolam	Versed
Beta-blockers	Propranolol	Inderal
Calcium-channel blockers	Amiodarone	Cordarone
	Diltiazem	Cardiazam
	Felodipine	Plendil
	Nicardipine	Cardene
	Nifedipine	Procardia
	Verapamil	Calan
Cholesterol-lowering drugs	Atorvastatin	Lipitor
	Cervivastatin	Baycol
	Lovastatin	Mevacor
	Simvastatin	Zocar

Signs of toxicity of local anesthetics with increasing blood levels (vary with individual patients)

- Metallic taste (copper penny)
- Numbness (circumoral, tongue)
- Lightheadedness
- Visual and auditory disturbances
- Slurred speech
- CNS excitement (restlessness, tremors)
- Drowsiness, loss of consciousness
- Convulsions
- CNS inhibition with respiratory arrest
- Cardiac arrest

Premedication

If premedication is felt to be necessary it may be given orally at home or on arrival to the office. The following are commonly used: diazepam (Valium) 5–10 mg, lorazepam (Ativan) 0.5–1 mg or alprazolam (Xanax) 0.5–1 mg. Alprazolam 0.5–1 mg given orally on arrival in the office (approximately 30 minutes before surgery) may reduce the required amount of conscious sedation by 50%. Clonidine is an antihypertensive that causes noticeable sedation without

Drugs commonly used in intravenous conscious sedation

impairing respiration. Klein believes that low-dose clonidine (0.1 mg) is an excellent anxiolytic for tumescent anesthesia. It also attenuates intraoperative hypertension and decreases the incidence of tachycardia associated with the use of epinephrine. Clonidine (0.1 mg) when combined with lorazepam 1 mg acts synergistically, reducing anxiety with minimal respiratory depression, and this combination has a long history of safe use in outpatient surgery. Neither drug interferes with the metabolism of lidocaine or other amide local anesthetics.

Premedication may also be given intramuscularly in the office (meperidine, promethazine, or midazolam). It must be borne in mind that the patient will need to stand for marking the leg if surface phlebectomy is to be performed.

Monitoring

The level of monitoring required in the office surgical setting is often determined by guidelines from the state licensing board. Physicians should check with their malpractice carrier to ensure coverage with their available level of monitoring.

It is always useful to have an intravenous (IV) access in place. Small Angiocaths™ (22- to 24-gauge) or butterflies (23- to 25-gauge) are adequate. The IV tubing used must have an injection port. Infusing a large volume of fluid early may lead to an uncomfortable patient with the need to urinate. A bedpan should be available for females and a urinal for males. Replacement fluids may not be necessary with tumescent anesthesia, since there is absorption of fluid through hypodermolysis.

Baseline vital signs should always be recorded. If any medications are given that may directly or indirectly produce hypoxia, the patient should be continuously monitored with a pulse oximeter and supplemental oxygen should be available. Intermittent blood pressures and pulse readings should be taken and documented. A continuous EKG is not essential, but may be required by state guidelines.

Intravenous conscious sedation

If IV conscious sedation is to be given, it should be started prior to the injection of any local anesthetic agent that is known to be painful. Once the operative area has been anesthetized with LA, there is minimal need for any further IV conscious sedation. Commonly used drugs in IV conscious sedation along with doses are listed in Table 13.7. Conscious sedation has been described as either "light" or "deep." Light sedation is when the level of consciousness is minimally depressed and the patient responds to verbal instructions and maintains a patent airway. In contrast, deep sedation refers to a state of depressed consciousness in which the patient may not respond to verbal commands and may require stimulation for adequate ventilation. Any time sedation goes beyond a "light" level, someone in the operative area should be assigned the sole responsibility of constantly monitoring the patient. An excellent review article on conscious sedation is available.

Drugs commonly used in intravenous conscious sedation
Morphine 5–10 mg (analgesic)
Meperidine (Demerol®) 25–100 mg (analgesic)
Fentanyl (Sublimaze®) 50–100 µg (analgesic)
Naloxone (Narcan®) 0.2–0.4 mg (opioid reversal)
Propofol (Diprivan®) 2.5–10 mg (rapid sedative hypnotic)
Promethazine (Phenergan®) 12.5–25 mg (antiemetic)
Diazepam (Valium®) 5–15 mg (anti-anxiety, anticonvulsant)
Midazolam (Versed®) 1–5 mg (anti-anxiety, amnesia)
Flumazenil (Romazicon®) 0.2 mg (benzodiazepine reversal)

Emergency supplies (Table 13.8)

It is wise to call the local 911 dispatching unit and ask for the estimated response time for the office location. For those comfortable with using endotracheal intubation, a laryngoscope with fresh batteries and an assortment (6–9 mm) of cuffed endotracheal tubes should be available. All emergency supplies must be kept in an easily accessible location. A fishing tackle box works well as an alternative to one of the commercially available emergency kits. All office personnel should know where these emergency supplies are kept and should be able to transport them wherever they may be needed.

Sudden cardiac arrest is the most common cause of death in the United States, accounting for an estimated 350 000 deaths annually. Life-threatening cardiac arrhythmias usually cause sudden cardiac arrest. Early defibrillation of ventricular tachycardia or ventricular fibrillation is necessary to resuscitate cardiac arrest victims, and survival depends directly on the time to defibrillation. Automated external defibrillators (AEDs) reduce the time to defibrillation, which leads to improved survival rates. All phlebologists should be aware of the clinical benefits of AEDs and the limited liability associated with their use, and should also consider the potential liability that could arise from failure to not have an AED. With the proven survival benefit provided by AEDs, it is likely that they will become a mandatory piece of safety equipment in all medical offices in the future.

Emergency supplies
IV fluids
Oxygen with mask/Ambu bag
Epinephrine
Atropine
Diphenhydramine (Benadryl®)
Ephedrine (vasopressor)
Nitroglycerin (Nitrostat®)
Diazepam IV (anticonvulsant)
Vasodilators (hydralazine, clonidine)
Aspirin

Summary

Phlebological treatments are now more effective than ever before, with streamlined outpatient methods allowing patients to return to their normal activities, usually within 24 hours. By effectively using appropriate anesthetic techniques, phlebologists can offer relatively pain-free treatments for venous disease in a pleasant office setting. As always, proper education and training, as well as attention to detail, will ensure the safety of the required anesthetic technique.

Bibliography

Breuninger H, Hobbach PS, Schimek F. Ropivacaine: an important agent for slow infusion and other forms of tumescent anesthesia. Dermatol Surg 1999; 25: 799–802.

Butterwick KJ, Goldman MP, Sriprachya-Anunt S. Lidocaine levels during the first two hours of infiltration of dilute anesthetic solution for tumescent liposuction: rapid versus slow delivery. Dermatol Surg 1999; 25: 681–5.

Christian M, Yeung L, Williams R, et al. Conscious sedation in dermatologic surgery. Dermatol Surg 2000; 26: 923–8.

Cohn M, Seiger E, Goldman S. Ambulatory phlebectomy using the tumescent technique for local anesthesia. Dermatol Surg 1995; 21: 315–18.

Coldiron B, Coleman WP III, Cox SE, et al. ASDS guidelines of care for tumescent liposuction. Dermatol Surg 2006; 32: 709–16.

Cousins MJ, Bridenbaugh PO, eds. Neural Blockade in Clinical Anesthesia and Management of Pain, 3rd edn. Philadelphia: Lippincott-Raven, 1998.

de Jong RH. Local Anesthetics. St Louis, MO: Mosby, 1994: 264–373.

England H, Weinberg P, Estes M. The automated external defibrillator. JAMA 2006; 295: 687–90.

Eriksson E, ed. Illustrated Handbook in Local Anesthesia, 2nd edn. London: WB Saunders, 1979: 10–23, 101–19.

Garde C. Ambulatory phlebectomy. Dermatol Surg 1995; 21: 628–30.

Klein JA. Tumescent technique for regional anesthesia permits lidocaine doses of 35 mg/kg for liposuction. J Dermatol Surg Oncol 1990; 16: 248–63.

Klein JA. Tumescent technique for local anesthesia improves safety in large volume liposuction. Plast Reconstr Surg 1993; 92: 1085–98.

Klein JA. Tumescent anesthesia for vein surgery. Venous Disease 2005; 1: 5–8.

Koay J, Orengo I. Application of local anesthesia in dermatologic surgery. Dermatol Surg 2002; 28: 143–8.

Lugo-Janer G, Padial M, Sáanchez JL. Less painful alternatives for local anesthesia. J Dermatol Surg Oncol 1993; 19: 237–40.

Miller RD, ed. Miller's Anesthesia, 6th edn. New York: Churchill Livingstone, 2005.

Moffitt DL, de Berker DAR, Kennedy CTK, Shutt LE. Assessment of ropivacaine as a local anesthetic for skin infiltration in skin surgery. Dermatol Surg 2001; 27: 437–40.

Moore DC. Regional Block: A Handbook for Use in Clinical Practice of Medicine/Surgery, 4th edn. Springfield, IL: Charles C Thomas, 1981: 3–49.

Nautias A, Kaplan B. Tumescent anesthesia for dermatologic surgery. Dermatol Surg 1998; 24: 755–8.

Neumann H. Ambulant minisurgical phlebectomy. J Dermatol Surg Oncol 1992; 18: 83–4.

Olivencia J. Local anesthesia for ambulatory phlebectomy. First Clinical Workshop of the American Society of Phlebectomy, Kansas City, October 1995.

Olivencia J. Ambulatory phlebectomy — a rare complication of local anesthetics: case report and literature review. Dermatol Surg 1996; 22: 53–5.

Onuma OC, Bearn PE, Khaira U, et al. The influence of effective analgesia and general anesthesia on patients' acceptance of day case varicose vein surgery. Phlebology 1993; 8: 29–31.

Ramesh S, Umeh H, Galland R. Day case varicose vein operations: patient suitability and satisfaction. Phlebology 1995; 10: 101–3.

Ricci S, Georgiev M. Office varicose vein surgery under local anesthesia. J Dermatol Surg Oncol 1992; 18: 55–8.

Ricci S, Georgiev M, Goldman MP, eds. Ambulatory Phlebectomy, 2nd edn. Boca Raton, FL: Taylor & Francis, 2005: 97–106.

Seager DJ, Simmons C. Local anesthesia in hair transplantation. Dermatol Surg 2002; 28: 320–8.

Staelens I, Van Der Stricht J. Complication rate of long stripping of the greater saphenous vein. Phlebology 1992; 7: 67–70.

Stoelting RK, Miller RD. Basics of Anesthesia, 5th edn. New York: Churchill Livingstone, 2007.

Thompson KD, Welykyj S, Massa MC. Antibacterial activity of lidocaine in combination with a bicarbonate buffer. J Dermatol Surg Oncol 1993; 19: 216–20.

Tretbar L. Local anesthesia for surgical treatment of varicose veins: my technique. First Clinical Workshop of the American Society of Phlebectomy, Kansas City, October 1995.

Vin F, Chleir F, Allaert FA. An ambulatory treatment of varicose veins associating surgical section and sclerotherapy of large saphenous veins. Dermatol Surg 1996; 22: 65–70.

A common but neglected problem

Epidemiological studies have found that the prevalence of leg ulceration in the adult population, either active or healed, is about 1%. Although a variety of etiologic factors can cause leg ulcers, the majority of leg ulcer patients have venous disease, and while chronic venous insufficiency has received less attention than arterial insufficiency, it is estimated to be 10 times more common. Despite the prevalence of venous ulcers, they are often neglected or managed inadequately. Patients may walk around for months or even years with just a local dressing. Too often, the emphasis may be placed on which ointment, cream, antibiotic, or enzyme should be used. The ulcers may be grafted only to recur.

Recognizing a venous ulcer

The classical presentation of a venous leg ulcer is an irregularly shaped partial-thickness wound with well-defined borders, surrounded by erythematous or hyperpigmented indurated skin (chronic lipodermatosclerosis) (Figure 1).

A yellow-white exudate is commonly observed. Venous ulcers vary in size and location, but are often found on the distal medial aspect of the lower leg ("gaiter" area). A lateral venous ulcer may be associated with small saphenous vein (SSV) insufficiency. Varicose veins are often present in the venous ulcer patient. Typically, there are telangiectatic veins in the medial ankle, so-called corona phlebectatica, indicative of chronic venous insufficiency. Edema of the ankle area is common, with a "champagne bottle deformity", with narrowing just above the bulk below the calf.

Other etiologies must be considered. Concomitant arterial insufficiency may be found in up to one-third of patients. Metabolic, neuropathic, neoplastic, vasculitic, infectious, hematologic, and collagen vascular diseases should be considered. However, if arterial insufficiency is ruled out and the patient has normal pinprick sensation in the face of a typical-appearing venous ulcer, a venous etiology will be found in 95% of cases.

The calf muscle pump

The calf muscle pump of the leg is the primary mechanism the body uses to return blood from the legs to the heart. The calf pump mechanism consists of the calf muscles, the deep venous compartment or pump chamber, a superficial compartment connecting the superficial veins to the deep veins (perforators), and an outflow tract (popliteal vein). Calf pump dysfunction may occur because of deep venous insufficiency (primary or post-thrombotic), deep venous obstruction, perforator insufficiency, superficial venous insufficiency, arteriovenous fistulas, neuromuscular dysfunction, or a combination of these factors. The result of calf pump dysfunction is a failure to lower venous pressure in the distal veins of the leg while walking, a condition referred to as ambulatory venous hypertension.

Macrocirculatory misconceptions

Structural venous abnormalities in any of the components of the calf pump can contribute to calf pump dysfunction. Nonetheless, the main factor in calf pump failure is usually

Venous leg ulcer. Image courtesy of Frank S. Frerichs.

venous insufficiency. A common misconception is that a venous leg ulcer is pathognomonic of a post-thrombotic syndrome. It is true that a deep vein thrombosis (DVT) may cause deep venous insufficiency and/or obstruction and lead to venous hypertension. However, it is not uncommon for venous leg ulcers to be due solely to superficial venous disease and/or perforator disease. In fact, superficial venous insufficiency was the primary contributor in at least 20% of venous ulcers in most series.[10,11] The common final pathway to venous ulceration is venous hypertension, whether the overload comes from superficial, perforator, deep vein, or combination disease.[6,9]

Microcirculatory abnormalities

It is unclear exactly how ambulatory venous hypertension causes ulceration. Chronic venous hypertension is associated with a number of microcirculatory abnormalities. These include extravasation of macromolecules (fibrinogen, albumin, macroglobulin, and others),[4] pericapillary fibrin cuff formation,[5] abnormalities of fibrinolysis,[5] leukocyte trapping and activation,[4] lymphatic microangiopathy, and abnormalities of the capillary network.[5]

In attempting to explain the pathogenesis of venous ulceration, Browse and Burnand put forth the fibrin cuff theory.[5] They suggested that pericapillary fibrin cuffs – typically but not exclusively found in patients with chronic venous insufficiency – act as an oxygen diffusion barrier. A number of publications have cast doubt on this premise.[6] A more recent theory involves leukocyte rheology.[7] With the reduction of capillary blood flow in venous hypertension, trains of leukocytes cause temporary plugging of capillaries. Glycoproteins cause leukocytes to become attached to capillary endothelium. These white cells become activated, releasing free radicals, proteolytic enzymes, and cytokines. Perhaps this chronic inflammatory state, if severe enough, leads to tissue damage and ulceration. Another hypothesis posits that fibrinogen and other macromolecules, which leak into the dermis as a result of venous hypertension and endothelial injury, "trap" growth factors and matrix proteins, and render them unavailable for the maintenance of tissue integrity and repair processes.[8] It is interesting to note that venous ulcer wound fluid, as distinguished from other acute wound fluid, inhibits in vitro proliferation of cells involved in wound healing such as fibroblasts, endothelial cells, and keratinocytes.[9] Bollinger states that the main factor in venous ulceration is focal microvascular ischemia secondary to the reduction of nutritive skin capillaries seen in chronic venous insufficiency.[5] Obviously, these theories are not mutually exclusive. As the pathogenesis of venous ulceration is elucidated, it is likely that therapeutic advances will occur.

History and physical examination

Details relating to the ulcer, such as its duration and past treatment, the presence and characteristics of exudate, and the presence of pain and factors that aggravate and alleviate the symptoms, should be sought. A history of similar lesions and their course and management is useful. In addition, a history of thromboembolic events, varicose veins, past vein treatment, tobacco abuse, arterial disease, diabetes, arthritis, ankle joint immobility, inflammatory bowel disease, and collagen vascular disease should be obtained. The patient's occupation and social situation should be determined.

Physical examination should include a careful inspection and palpation of the legs, from the foot to the groin, for varicose veins. The suprapubic area should also be inspected for varicosities, which might represent collateral bypass of an old iliofemoral thrombosis (Figure 14.2).

The patient should be examined for signs of chronic venous insufficiency, such as ankle flare, eczema, hyperpigmentation, induration, and atrophie blanche. Ankle and calf diameters should be recorded for both legs. The characteristics of edema (pitting vs nonpitting) should be noted.

The ulcer(s) size, base, appearance, and location, in addition to the condition of the surrounding skin, should be described. The presence and characteristics of exudate and signs of true tissue infection are noted. Note that acute lipodermatosclerosis, characterized by an erythematous tender area of induration (Figure 14.3), is commonly mistaken for cellulitis. It is an inflammatory condition due to venous insufficiency, which does not cause fever and is unresponsive to antibiotics.

Signs of arterial insufficiency (cool skin, loss of extremity hair, shiny and atrophic skin, and pallor on leg elevation) should be noted. Arterial pulses should be palpated. If there is suspicion of arterial insufficiency, an ankle–brachial index (ABI; systolic pressure at the ankle divided by that at the brachial artery; normal > 0.9) should be done. Note that the ABI is unreliable in assessing arterial insufficiency in diabetes and other conditions where there may be arterial calcification. In such cases, toe pressures are more reliable. Ankle mobility and gait should be evaluated. Peripheral sensation should be checked.

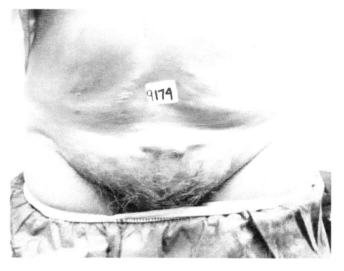

Suprapubic or abdominal varices indicate iliofemoral obstruction. (Image courtesy of James Altizer MD)

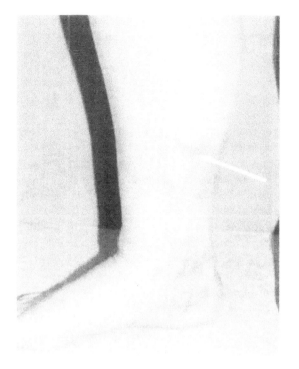

Acute lipodermatosclerosis (arrow). (Image courtesy of Helane S Fronek MD)

Elucidation of underlying abnormal hemodynamics

It is important to define the underlying abnormal hemodynamics of a venous ulcer patient because of the implications for treatment (see "Individualized treatment" below). In addition to a history and physical examination, a functional and anatomic test should be used to obtain a complete picture of the venous abnormality. Duplex ultrasound yields both anatomic and functional information about the venous system of the legs. Investigation of the great saphenous vein (GSV), SSV, perforating veins, femoral vein, popliteal vein, and the deep veins of the calf should be done. Plethysmographic tests, such as photoplethysmography and air plethysmography, are functional tests that can be used to evaluate venous reflux, calf pump function, and venous outflow. Utilizing tourniquets to occlude superficial veins, these plethysmographic tests can help assess the likelihood of hemodynamic improvement following treatment of superficial and perforator vein incompetence in a patient who also has deep vein disease. Invasive tests are generally not necessary. Although previously thought to be due entirely to post thrombotic changes, venous ulceration is much more frequently the result of treatable abnormalities within the superficial and perforator segments of the venous system.

Compression as the cornerstone of treatment

All ambulatory patients with uninfected venous ulceration require compression treatment. Such treatment should be sustained compression that produces a pressure gradient (highest at the ankle). Bandages (elastic and inelastic) and stockings have been used. Inelastic compression devices such as the CircAid (CircAid Medical Products, Inc., San Diego, CA) have also been used. Generally, the adage is true that compression bandaging obtains a result and compression stockings maintain the result. In the decongestive phase, compression bandaging is best done with inelastic "short-stretch" bandages. Expertise in applying a short stretch bandage is required. Short-stretch bandages may be left on for several days (up to a week). Early in treatment, until exudate and edema diminish, it may be necessary to re-apply the bandages more frequently. In the face of concomitant arterial insufficiency, one must exercise considerable caution: it is imperative that any compression exert a low resting pressure (inelastic compression). If arterial insufficiency is severe, compression of any type may be contraindicated.

Examples of short-stretch bandages are Unna's paste bandage and Comprilan (BSN-JOBST, Inc., Rutherford College, NC). ACE bandages are inadequate as a treatment of venous ulceration. Prescription compression stockings can be used in the maintenance phase of treatment. Generally, calf length stockings are used with 30–40 or 40–50 mmHg. It is easier for some patients to apply a zippered stocking over a nylon liner (Jobst UlcerCARE; BSN-JOBST, Inc., Rutherford College, NC) or to superimpose two 20–30 mmHg stockings (yielding 40 mmHg). Consider intermittent pneumatic compression in patients who do not respond to standard compression measures and in patients who are not ambulatory.

Compression leads to increased venous flow, decreased pathologic reflux while walking, and an increased ejection volume with activation of the calf pump. Tissue pressure is increased, which favors resorption of edema fluid. In order to achieve maximum benefit from compression, the patient needs to ambulate. A regular regimen of at least 30 minutes of daily walking is extremely beneficial.

Wound care

Local wound care is a matter of clinical judgment. Debridement can be accomplished with surgical instruments, with topical enzymatic agents, and by autolytic debridement with occlusive dressings. Generally, it is appropriate to choose the least invasive methods first. Normal (0.9%) saline can be used for wound cleansing. Wounds should be covered with a semipermeable dressing or non-adherent gauze. If there is a lot of exudate, a highly absorptive dressing should be chosen. It should be remembered that good compression is useful in reducing noninfectious exudate. Moisture-retentive dressings frequently cause a malodorous yellow discharge that many patients mistakenly think represents infection. A foam pad worn over the dressing and under the compression bandaging increases local compression and helps reduce local venous hypertension. Topical antibiotics are generally not used. In fact, contact dermatitis to topical antibiotics commonly develops in patients with chronic venous insufficiency. However, one study found that venous ulcer patients treated with silver sulfadiazine cream plus compression healed significantly faster than a group treated with compression alone.[24] In the face of an acute weeping dermatitis, one should consider advising leg elevation and the use of saline soaks followed by a mid-potency cortisone cream. If there is a concern about cortisone sensitization, a short course of oral corticosteroids could be considered. Petrolatum or other bland emollients can be used on surrounding dry skin. If true tissue infection is suspected, cultures should be taken and treatment begun with systemic antibiotics.

If a venous ulcer patient has hemodynamically significant superficial venous disease, either isolated or in combination with perforator or deep vein disease, important hemodynamic improvement will be obtained by treating the venous insufficiency and the long-term prognosis will thereby be greatly improved. Treatment may include surgery, endovenous ablative techniques, or sclerotherapy. An important exception exists in the face of significant deep venous obstruction, where the superficial varices may act as an important outflow tract. Removal of superficial veins in this situation is contraindicated. However, a study found that less than 10% of patients with deep venous obstruction had a significant decrease in venous outflow fraction when superficial veins were occluded.[25] These authors suggested that deep vein collaterals may be more important than superficial collaterals following significant deep vein obstruction. Outflow measurements using a variety of plethysmographic techniques may be helpful in determining which patients are relying on superficial veins for venous outflow.

The hemodynamic significance of perforators in chronic venous insufficiency remains controversial.[25] The development of subfascial endoscopic ligation has significantly improved the surgical treatment of incompetent medial calf perforators,[26] although failure of ulcer healing or recurrence of ulceration after endoscopic perforator ligation has ranged from 2.5% to 22%.[27] A potential limitation of this technique is the difficulty in accessing perimalleolar perforators. One study found that 50% of incompetent perforators within 10 cm of the sole of the foot, identified preoperatively by duplex ultrasound, were missed at subfascial endoscopy.[27] More recently, thermal ablation of perforators has been accomplished using radiofrequency or laser energy.

Deep venous reconstruction should only be done as a last resort, in the face of intractable pain or ulceration or impairment of function in spite of conservative measures and correction of any superficial venous insufficiency. The fundamental treatment of deep venous insufficiency is lifelong compression. However, sclerotherapy of periulcer varices and perforators can significantly improve local venous hemodynamics and can speed ulcer healing.[28] It is generally accepted that significant insufficiency within the superficial venous system should be corrected if possible. Also, studies have demonstrated that

some incompetent deep veins normalize following treatment of incompetent superficial veins, presumably as a result of reducing load on the deep veins.[29]

Patients should be instructed to maintain a normal weight and to avoid smoking. Nutritional deficiencies should be corrected. Regular brisk walking, preferably five times per week for at least 30 minutes per walk, should be strongly encouraged. Long periods of sitting and standing and extremely hot baths should be avoided. It is helpful to have the patient periodically elevate their leg above heart level and to raise the foot of their bed with 3-inch blocks. Manual lymphatic drainage, performed by trained therapists, can reduce the edema of chronic venous insufficiency. Physical therapy can improve ankle joint mobility, which has been shown to reduce ulcer duration and recurrence. Diuretics generally are not used. Pentoxifylline seems to reduce leukocyte trapping and may improve venous ulcer healing when used in conjunction with compression therapy.[30]

If a patient does not respond to appropriate therapy, the physician should question the adequacy of compression and/or patient compliance. The diagnosis needs to be questioned, and the possibility of tissue infection or malignancy should be considered. Obtaining a biopsy of the ulcer edge is indicated at that point.

A significant social and economic burden is caused by chronic venous insufficiency. Newer methods of investigation have led to an improvement in our understanding of the pathophysiology of venous disease. Compression should serve as the cornerstone of treatment in venous ulcers. However, superficial and/or perforator disease may be the underlying cause of venous ulceration in a significant percentage of patients, and treatment of these patients with surgery, endovenous ablation, and/or sclerotherapy can greatly improve their prognosis. Thus, duplex ultrasound examination must be performed in every patient in order to define the underlying abnormalities of the venous system and any associated diseases to form a rational, individualized management plan for the patient with venous ulceration.

1. Callam MJ, Ruckley CV, Harper DR, et al. Chronic ulceration of the leg: extent of the problem and provision of care. BMJ 1985; 290: 1855–6.
2. Widmer LK. Peripheral venous disorders: prevalence and socio-medical importance. Observations in 4529 apparently healthy persons. Basel Study III. Bern: Hans Huber, 1978: 43–50.
3. Baker SR, Stacey MC, Jopp-McKay AG, et al. Epidemiology of chronic venous ulcers. Br J Surg 1991; 78: 864–7.

4. Scriven JM, Hartshorne T, Bell PRF, et al. Single-visit venous ulcer assessment clinic: the first year. Br J Surg 1997; 84: 334–6.

5. O'Donnell TF Jr. Chronic venous insufficiency: an overview of epidemiology, classification, and anatomic considerations. Semin Vasc Surg 1988; 1: 60–5.

6. Goldman MP, Fronek A. The Alexander House Group. Consensus paper on venous leg ulcer. J Dermatol Surg Oncol 1992; 18: 592–602.

7. Bass A, Chayen D, Weinmann EE, Ziss M. Lateral venous ulcer and short saphenous vein insufficiency. J Vasc Surg 1997; 25: 654–7.

8. Cornwall JV, Lewis JD. Leg ulcers revisited. Br J Surg 1983; 70: 681.

9. Burton CS. Successful leg ulcer management. Annual Meeting of the American Academy of Dermatology, 1993.

10. Hanrahan LM, Araki CT, Rodriguez AA, et al. Distribution of valvular incompetence in patients with venous stasis ulceration. J Vasc Surg 1991; 13: 805–11.

11. Hoare MC, Nicolaides AN, Miles CR, et al. The role of primary varicose veins in venous ulceration. Surgery 1982; 92: 450–3.

12. Darke SG, Penfold C. Venous ulceration and saphenous ligation. Eur J Vasc Surg 1992; 6: 4–9.

13. Zimmet SE. Leg ulcers. J Am Acad Dermatol 1992; 27: 487–8.

14. Falanga V, Eaglstein WH. The "trap" hypothesis of venous ulceration. Lancet 1993; 341: 1006–8.

15. Browse NL, Burnand KG. The cause of venous ulceration. Lancet 1982; ii: 243–5.

16. Coleridge Smith PD, Thomas P, Scurr JH, et al. Causes of venous ulceration: a new hypothesis? BMJ 1988; 296: 1726–7.

17. Stibe E, Cheatle TR, Coleridge Smith PD, et al. Liposclerotic skin: a diffusion block or perfusion problem? Phlebology 1990; 5: 231–6.

18. Cheatle TR, McMullin GM, Farrah J, et al. Skin damage in chronic venous insufficiency: Does an oxygen diffusion barrier really exist? J R Soc Med 1990; 83: 48–9.

19. Michel CC. Oxygen diffusion in oedematous tissue and through pericapillary fibrin cuffs. Phlebology 1990; 5: 223?30.

20. Claudy AL, Mirshahi M, Suria C, et al. Detection of undegraded fibrin and tumor necrosis factor α in venous leg ulcers. J Am Acad Dermatol 1991; 25: 623–7.

21. Bucalo B, Eaglstein WH, Falanga V. The effect of chronic wound fluid on cell proliferation in vitro. J Invest Dermatol 1989; 92: 539.

22. Bollinger A. A rejected letter to the editors of The Lancet and the need for angiologists to prove their usefulness. Vasa 1993; 22: 361–3.

23. Partsch H. Contributions Towards Compression Therapy. Neuwied: Lohmann, 1990: 11–12.

24. Bishop JB, Phillips LG, Mustoe TA, et al. A prospective random-ized evaluator-blinded trial of two potential wound healing agents for the treatment of venous stasis ulcers. J Vasc Surg 1992; 16: 251–7.

25. Labropoulos N, Voltea N, Leon M, et al. The role of venous out-flow obstruction in patients with chronic venous insufficiency. Arch Surg 1997; 132: 46–51.

26. Bergan J. Endoscopic subfascial perforator vein interruption. In: Goldman MP, Bergan JJ, eds. Ambulatory Treatment of Venous Disease: An Illustrative Guide. St Louis, MO: Mosby, 1996: 173–8.

27. Pierik EGJM, van Urk H, Wittens CHA. Efficacy of subfascial endoscopy in eradicating perforating veins of the lower leg and its relation with venous ulcer healing. J Vasc Surg 1997; 26: 255–9.

28. Queral LA, Criado FJ, Lilly MP, Rudolphi D. The role of scle-rotherapy as an adjunct to Unna's boot for treating venous ulcers: a prospective study. J Vasc Surg 1990; 11: 572–5.

29. Walsh JC, Bergan JJ, Beeman S, Comer TP. Femoral venous reflux abolished by greater saphenous stripping. Ann Vasc Surg 1994; 8:566-70.

30. Dormandy JA. Pharmacologic treatment of venous leg ulcers. J Cardiovasc Pharmacol 1995; 25(Suppl): S61–5.

Thrombophlebitis is a potentially life-threatening complication of many medical conditions and surgical procedures. Epidemiological data have shown that in a given practice of 10 000 surgical patients, 39 cases of venous thromboembolism (VTE) with 11 associated deaths from this cause will be recognized per year. In fact, the incidence may be significantly higher, since many cases go undiagnosed. One in nine people will develop deep vein thrombosis (DVT) before the age of 80 and clinically recognized embolic disease accounts for one in 20 deaths after age 50. In women, embolic disease accounts for the majority of non-abortive, pregnancy-related maternal mortality in the United States.[1,2] These statistics make it important to have a high degree of clinical suspicion when signs and symptoms of this disorder are present.

Superficial thrombophlebitis (STP) implies both inflammation and thrombus formation within a superficial vein.[3] It is most commonly seen in the lower extremity in association with varicose veins. Its course is usually benign and self-limiting; however, a thorough diagnostic evaluation Is necessary in patients with suspected STP, since they may have concomitant occult DVT.[4] Virchow's triad, consisting of venous stasis, endothelial damage, and hypercoagulability, is important in the development of STP. Often, there is a history of trauma to the vein or a decrease in activity level, such as with travel. Patients present with pain and localized tenderness over a firm reticular or varicose vein. Less often, telangiectasias may be involved. Diffuse leg pain and edema are not uncommon, although the findings are usually more localized.

Physical examination is helpful in ruling out other conditions that may be confused with STP. For example, diffuse erythema and swelling beyond the course of the vein could suggest cellulitis or lymphangitis. The presence of fever, tender lymphadenopathy and an elevated white blood cell count may favor these diagnoses. Musculoskeletal and neurologic causes of pain and tenderness, such as fibromyalgia or myositis, also need to be considered. Duplex ultrasound (DUS) is helpful in the evaluation of patients with SVT, and can also determine if DVT is present, as patients with STP and associated varicose veins have a 4–20% incidence of concomitant DVT. Even more important is the fact that patients with

STP without varicose veins have a 40% chance of concomitant DVT. Recurrent or migratory STP should prompt an evaluation for underlying malignancy, inherited coagulopathies (thrombophilias), or other hypercoagulable states.

Treatment includes graduated compression (a class I or II stocking is easiest for the patient), and frequent ambulation. Nonsteroidal anti-inflammatory drugs (NSAIDs) may be used for pain, with resolution usually occurring within 2–3 weeks. Bed rest is contraindicated. Fortunately, STP is usually a benign and short-term condition. Caution must be taken if duplex ultrasound shows the thrombus to be within a few centimeters of a deep vein (saphenofemoral or saphenopopliteal junction, SFJ or SPJ), in which case urgent ligation, thrombolysis, or low-molecular–weight heparin may be indicated.

While STP is usually benign and short-term, DVT can cause significant morbidity and chronic venous insufficiency, as well as fatal pulmonary embolism (PE).[5] DVT is often first noticed as a sensation of "pulling" or "fullness" in the posterior aspect of the lower leg, although the onset of pain may be acute and severe. In pregnancy and the postpartum period, the left leg is involved more often. Symptoms generally worsen with ambulation. Calf tenderness and a positive "Homan's sign" (pain with dorsiflexion of the foot) are not pathognomonic and are generally unreliable in confirming the diagnosis of DVT.

Diagnosis of DVT

Certain historical risk factors can increase the clinical suspicion of DVT. These risk factors are classified as either major or minor risks. Major risk factors include:

> age > 60
> history of prior DVT or PE
> prolonged immobility >72 hours/paralysis
> malignancy
> severe infection or sepsis
> inherited coagulopathies (thrombophilias)
> other hypercoagulable states
> myocardial infarction
> heart failure, decompensated
> central venous access

Minor risk factors include:

obesity (body mass index, BMI > 30)
heart failure, compensated
trauma
pregnancy or postpartum period
varicose veins
oral contraceptive use
hormone replacement therapy
recent surgery or travel

In general, patients are considered to be at low risk for DVT If they are under age 40 with one or no minor risk factors. Those under the age of 40 with more than one minor risk factor – or those over 40 with any risk factor – are considered to be at moderate to high risk for the development of DVT. Patients at moderate to high risk should be considered for DVT prophyxis prior to surgery. This can be accomplished with intermittent pneumatic compression stockings, pharmaceutical prophylaxis, or both.

A helpful screening approach to the diagnosis of DVT is D-dimer testing.[6] D-dimer levels reflect the amount of lysed, crosslinked fibrin and may be a useful diagnostic marker in patients with clinically suspected DVT. Enzyme-linked immunosorbent assay (ELISA) or rapid quantitative ELISA have both been shown to have a very high negative predictive value for DVT and PE. A negative result is as helpful in ruling out a DVT as a negative lower extremity duplex examination and as helpful in ruling out a PE as a negative perfusion lung scan or CT scan. Unfortunately, D-dimer is elevated by a variety of nonthrombotic disorders, including recent surgery, hemorrhage, trauma, pregnancy, and malignancy. Its use, therefore, may be limited in these clinical settings.

Most vascular laboratories offer duplex ultrasound examination as the diagnostic test of choice. More than any other noninvasive diagnostic tool, duplex ultrasound has emerged as the most effective, cost-efficient, and reliable method to evaluate the peripheral venous system. This test, however, is very operator-dependent and thus prone to false-negative and -positive results. With duplex ultrasound imaging, the popliteal and femoral veins can be visualized and thrombi directly seen. The paired axial veins of the distal lower extremity (anterior tibial, posterior tibial, and peroneal veins) may not be as easily visualized, and require more expertise on the part of the sonographer. When ultrasound fails to confirm a suspected DVT, magnetic resonance venography (MRV) may be helpful.[7] MRV is as accurate as contrast venography in visualizing DVT, can detect thrombi in pelvic veins that are not well visualized on DUS, and may provide a diagnosis if DVT is not present. Contrast venography has fallen out of favor, since it requires injection of contrast material that may cause an allergic reaction or renal damage. When definitive testing is not immediately available and the likelihood of DVT is high, the patient should be immediately fully anticoagulated while awaiting a definitive test. If a coagulopathy is suspected, appropriate blood tests should be drawn before anticoagulation is instituted.

When treated, fewer than 5% of DVTs progress to PE, with

a 1% mortality. If unrecognized, 25–60% of DVTs progress to PE, with a 15% mortality rate. Diagnosis is often accomplished with ventilation–perfusion ratio ($\dot{V}/\dot{Q}$) scanning, but pulmonary angiography may be used as well. Computed tomography (CT) scanning is evolving as the contemporary screening method of choice. A high index of suspicion for PE is necessary, since signs may be subtle. Classic findings include pleuritic chest pain, hemoptysis, shortness of breath, tachycardia, tachypnea, and a decreased oxygen saturation.

Thrombolysis should be considered in all patients who have thrombus in the deep venous system, unless contraindications exist, as thrombolysis is the only form of therapy that dissolves a clot and therefore may protect venous valvular function. However, based on the available evidence, the American College of Chest Physicians does not currently recommend the routine use of intravenous or catheter-directed thrombolysis in patients with DVT, except in the case of limb-threatening phlegmasia.[9]

Heparin therapy increases thrombolysis by activating antithrombin. It is a bulky molecule that does not cross the placenta, is not secreted in breast milk, and is therefore safe in pregnant and lactating women. Unfractionated heparin (UFH) is often administered in a dose of 500 U/kg/day to maintain the activated partial thromboplastin time (aPTT) at 2–2.5 times the baseline value. The following is an effective protocol:

Heparin 10 000 units IV push.
Initial infusion approximately 20 units/kg/h.
Adjust heparin at 6–8 h intervals to maintain aPTT 2–2.5 times baseline value.
Start warfarin 10 mg/day on second day, combining IV heparin and oral warfarin for at least 4 days.
Follow prothrombin time (PT) daily and adjust warfarin to maintain the International Normalized Ratio (INR) at 2.0–3.0.
Continue warfarin for 6–12 months, monitoring INR carefully.

Warfarin blocks vitamin K and the vitamin K-dependent coagulation factors II, VII, IX, and X. Controversy still exists regarding the duration of warfarin therapy and the indications for lifelong anticoagulation, as well as the indications for evaluation of hypercoagulability. Warfarin is teratogenic and should not be given to pregnant women. It may cause nasal hypoplasia and skeletal defects with first-trimester exposure and intracranial bleeding with second- and third-trimester exposures. It is safe, however, when used in breastfeeding mothers.

With proper dosing, several low-molecular-weight heparin (LMWH) products have been found to be safer, more effective, and less costly than UFH for both prophylaxis and treatment of DVT and PE.[10] It is neither necessary nor useful to monitor aPTT when using LMWH. These products are most active in the tissues, and do not exert most of their effects on

Treatment of the leg

Hypercoagulability

Prevalence of thrombophilias in the general population, in patients with a first venous thromboembolism, and in thrombophilic families

Hypercoagulable state	General population	Patients with first VTE	Thrombophilic families
Factor V Leiden	3–7%	20%	50%
Prothrombin 20210 mutation	1–3%	6%	18%
Antithrombin deficiency	0.02%	1%	4–8%
Protein C deficiency	0.2–0.4%	3%	6–8%
Protein S deficiency	NA	1–2%	3–13%
Hyperhomocysteinemia	5–10%	10–25%	NA
Antiphospholipid antibodies	0–7%	5–15%	NA

NA, not available.

of some of these thrombophilias in different patient populations is shown in Table 15.1.

Although many phlebologists initially limit the scope of their practice to the treatment of minor superficial venous disease, it is advisable to have a working knowledge of the more serious venous disorders in order to accurately diagnose patients who present with them and to offer specialty expertise in the full range of phlebological conditions.

References

1. Kaunitz AM, Hughes JM, Grimes DA, et al. Causes of maternal mortality in the United States. Obstet Gynecol 1985; 65: 605–12.
2. Nima, JG. Obstetric embolic disease. The Female Patient 2002; 27(3): 12–14.
3. Markovic MD, Lotina SI, Davidovic LB, et al. [Acute superficial thrombophlebitis – modern diagnosis and therapy.] Srp Arh Celok Lek 1997; 125: 261–6.
4. Bounmeaux H, Reber-Wasem MA. Superficial thrombophlebitis and deep vein thrombosis: a controversial association. Arch Intern Med 1997; 157: 1822–4.
5. Tovey C, Wyatt S. Diagnosis, investigation and management of deep vein thrombosis. BMJ 2003; 326: 1180–4.
6. Stein PD, Hull RD, Patel KC, et al. D-dimer for the exclusion of acute venous thrombosis and pulmonary embolism. A systematic review. Ann Intern Med 2004; 140: 589–602.
7. Carpenter JP, Holland GA, Baum RA, et al. Magnetic resonance venography for the detection of deep venous thrombosis: comparison with contrast venography and duplex Doppler ultrasonography. J Vasc Surg 1993; 18: 734–41.
8. Hirsh J, Hoak J. Management of deep vein thrombosis and pulmonary embolism. A statement for health professionals. Council on Thrombosis (in consultation with the Council on Cardiovascular Radiology), American Heart Association. Circulation 1996; 93: 2212–45.
9. Buller H, Kucher N, Kiptmueller E, et al. Antithrombotic therapy for venous thromboembolic disease: the Seventh ACCP Conference on Antithrombotic and Thrombolytic Therapy. Chest 2004; 126: 401S–28S.
10. Haver KE. Low-molecular-weight heparin in the treatment of deep venous thrombosis. West J Med 1998; 169: 240–4.
11. Levine MN, Hirsh J, Gent M, et al. Optimal duration of oral anticoagulation therapy: a randomized trial comparing four weeks with three months of warfarin in patients with proximal deep vein thrombosis. Thromb Haemost 1995; 74: 606–11.
12. Duguid DL. Oral anticoagulant therapy for venous thromboembolism. N Engl J Med 1997; 336: 433–4.
13. Kearon C, Gent M, Hirsh J, et al. A comparison of three months of anticoagulation with extended anticoagulation for a first episode of idiopathic venous thromboembolism. N Engl J Med 1999; 340: 901–7.
14. Schulman S, Granqvist S, Holmstrom M, et al. The duration of oral anticoagulant therapy after a second episode of venous thromboembolism. The Duration of Anticoagulation Trial Study Group. N Engl J Med 1997; 336: 393–8.
15. Partsch H, Kechavarz B, Kohn H, Mostbeck A. The effect of mobilization of patients during treatment of thromboembolic disorders with low-molecular-weight heparin. Int Angiol 1997; 16: 189–92.
16. Prandoni P, Lensing AW, Prins MH, et al. Below-knee elastic compression stockings to prevent the post-thrombotic syndrome. A randomized, controlled trial. Ann Intern Med 2004; 141: 249–56.
17. Morris RJ, Woodcock JP. Evidence-based compression: prevention of stasis and deep vein thrombosis. Ann Surg 2004; 239: 162–71.
18. Barger AP, Hurley R. Evaluation of the hypercoagulable state. Whom to screen, how to test and treat. Postgrad Med 2000; 108(4): 59–66.
19. Deitcher SR, Gomes MPV. Hypercoagulable states. Cleveland Clinic Disease Management Project. http://www.clevelandclinicmeded.com/medicalpubs/diseasemanagement/hematology/hyperco/hyperco.htm.

The medical literature in the field of phlebology has been difficult to use in an effective fashion – in part due to the complexity in both venous anatomy and pathology, but also due to the absence of a classification system that distinguishes the forms and severity of venous disease being treated. In an attempt to allow a clear description of the type of venous disease being discussed – and thus to compare "apples with apples" – the CEAP classification was established.

The letter "C" is based on clinical findings, usually seen on physical examination (Figure 16.1):

C_0 = no visible venous disease

C_1 = telangiectatic or reticular veins

C_2 = varicose veins

C_3 = edema

C_4 = skin changes without ulceration

C_5 = skin changes with healed ulceration

C_6 = skin changes with active ulceration

More than one number may be assigned if the patient has several findings on clinical examination. After the numeric subscript, the letter "a" is assigned if the patient is asymptomatic or "s" if the patient experiences symptoms. Lastly, an additional number may follow the "s" to denote the severity of the symptom. The clinical disability scores for chronic venous insufficiency are:

0 = a patient who is asymptomatic, and thus has no disability

1 = a patient who is symptomatic but can function without a support device

2 = a patient who can work an 8-hour day only with a support device

3 = a patient who is unable to work even with a support device

The "E" stands for etiology, with subscript "c" for congenital disease, "p" for primary disease (not due to another cause), or "s" for secondary venous disease, usually due to prior deep vein thrombosis.

The "A" refers to the anatomic findings, usually based on duplex ultrasound examination. The options are as follows:

Superficial veins (A_s)

1. Telangiectasias or reticular veins
2. Great saphenous vein – above the knee
3. Great saphenous vein – below the knee
4. Small saphenous vein
5. Nonsaphenous

Deep veins (A_d)

6. Inferior vena cava
7. Common iliac
8. Internal iliac
9. External iliac
10. Pelvic: gonadal, broad ligament, etc.
11. Common femoral
12. Deep femoral
13. Femoral (between the groin and the knee)
14. Popliteal
15. Crural: anterior tibial, posterior tibial, peroneal
16. Muscular: gastrocnemius, soleus, etc.

Perforating veins (A_p)

17. Thigh
18. Calf

The "P" refers to the pathophysiologic component, with subscript "r" for reflux, "o" for obstruction, or "r,o" for both reflux and obstruction.

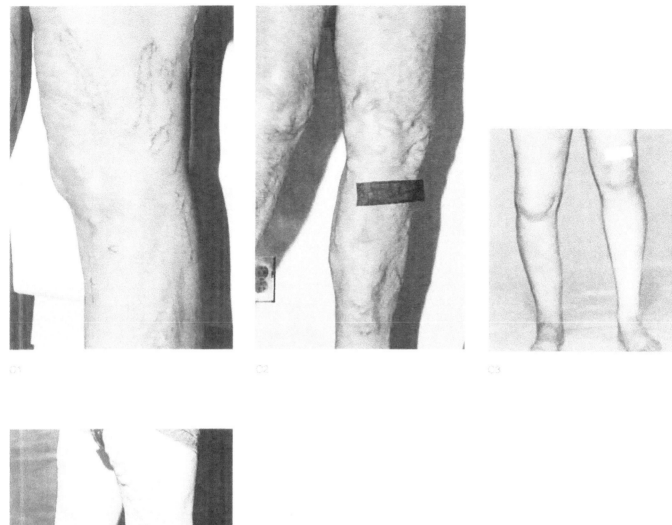

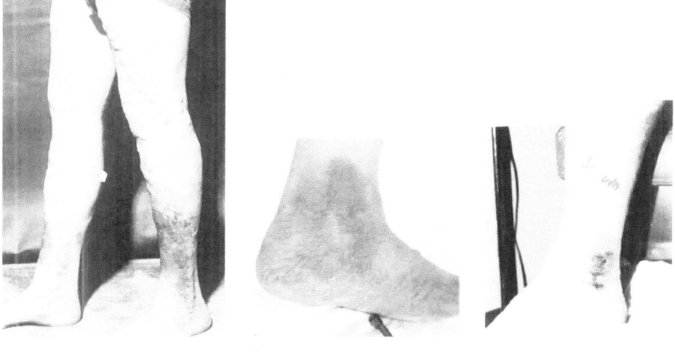

Clinical findings (C) in the CEAP classification. (Images courtesy of Helane S. Fronek, MD)

A classification of

$$C_{1,2,4,5\ s-2}\ E_p\ A_{s-1,2,3\ p-17,18}\ P_r$$

indicates a symptomatic ($C_{...s}$) patient with primary (E_p) telangiectasias, varicose veins, active skin changes, and a healed venous ulcer ($C_{1,2,4,5}$). There is reflux (P_r) in the telangiectasias and reticular veins, the great saphenous vein above and below the knee, and perforating veins in the thigh and calf ($A_{s-1,2,3\ p-17,18}$). This patient's symptoms are severe enough to require a compression stocking in order to function during an 8-hour working day ($C_{...s-2}$).

The use of the CEAP classification routinely in patient records and in the medical literature allows the efficacy of treatments to be compared and the progress of patients to be followed in an intelligent and meaningful way. Implementation of this classification is an easily achieved goal, and all phlebologists are encouraged to use this tool in their daily practice.

The practice of phlebology may be initiated as a full- or part-time endeavor, as many physicians who treat patients with venous disease also practice in another specialty, such as primary care, dermatology, surgery, or interventional radiology. The physician's primary specialty may influence which of the various treatment modalities – compression, exercise, sclerotherapy, surgery, and laser – are incorporated into the practice. Before starting such a practice, sufficient thought should be given to the spectrum of venous disease, treatment options, and complications of any treatment undertaken. As with all medical education, appropriate courses should be taken, and hands-on experience is advised. Since no residency-level training exists in this field, developing a relationship with an experienced phlebologist can be helpful as new situations are encountered in the practice. The American College of Phlebology (ACP) continues to develop educational opportunities to service the needs of its growing membership, and preceptorships, fellowships, and a board-certification examination and review courses are planned.

Education begins with learning the anatomy, physiology, pathophysiology, and differential diagnoses. All available treatment options, including their short- and long-term outcomes, should be considered. Seminars and courses in the field of phlebology introduce the newcomer to experienced practitioners, and preceptorships and periods of observation may also be arranged. Medical literature in many languages with both historical and current coverage of experimental and clinical studies exists, and may be found in the following journals: *Dermatologic Surgery* (formerly *Journal of Dermatologic Surgery and Oncology*), *Phlebology*, and the *Journal of Vascular Surgery*. The *Venous Digest* provides a monthly overview of phlebology literature and is available online. Several textbooks provide excellent coverage for the specialty of phlebology The reader is referred to the bibliography at the end of this chapter.

Staffing for a phlebology practice requires a team approach and should include professionals to help gather historical and physical information, perform physical and ultrasound examinations, assist with and perform various procedures, apply dressings, provide patient education, and facilitate patient flow. Roles can be filled by medical assistants, ultrasonographers, nurses, or physician's assistants. Having a nurse or physician's assistant who also performs sclerotherapy and who can assist with surgical and endovenous procedures facilitates patient care and provides more flexibility for the practice.

The practice of phlebology exposes physician and staff to the possibility of needlesticks and bloodborne pathogens. A thorough understanding of Occupational Safety and Health Administration (OSHA) guidelines and postexposure protocols is necessary. As with all medical practices, handwashing, gloves, and protective eye gear are important considerations, and hepatitis B vaccination is advised. Health Insurance Portability and Accountability Act (HIPAA) guidelines must also be followed.

In order to properly evaluate the phlebology patient, several diagnostic tools are necessary after a history and physical examination have been performed. An indispensable piece of medical equipment that has emerged in the past few years is duplex ultrasound imaging with Doppler spectral analysis and color flow. Duplex examinations range from screening for initial venous insufficiency assessment, to therapeutic guidance, and, finally, to long-term assessment. Procedures such as duplex ultrasound-directed sclerotherapy add significantly to the efficacy of sclerotherapy, whether with liquid or foamed sclerosants. Ultrasound imaging is also an integral part of endothermal ablative procedures for the great and small saphenous vein systems. The physician phlebologist should attain proficiency in ultrasound examination, as this provides essential information regarding the patient's pathology.

Where medical photography was once considered to belong in the hands of a few talented people with both expensive equipment and a vast knowledge base required to be proficient in 35 mm photography, and cataloguing and storage of the thousands of slides was a logistical problem, today digital photography facilitates both the acquisition and storage of images.

Pretreatment, treatment in progress, and post-treatment images are important for any and all insurance claims, and also allow both physician and patient to accurately assess the response to treatment. There are several considerations involved in selecting the process to be incorporated into the office.

Camera

In selecting a camera, the first question concerns the optimal number of megapixels of the camera's sensor. With manufacturers releasing new products every few months, the answer to this question changes rapidly. However, there are some basic principles that will assist the novice photographer in making an appropriate decision. In general, 4 megapixels are the minimum necessary for phlebology, and outstanding results can be obtained with 5–10 megapixels. Products in current use that have been shown to produce excellent images include:

- Panasonic FZ-30 (8 megapixels) with 12× optical zoom and image stabilization, ("point and shoot")
- Sony DSC V3 (7.2 megapixels) with 5× optical zoom
- Sony DSC R1 (10 megapixels) with 5× optical zoom
- Canon Rebel and EOS series DSLRs (single lens reflex (SLR) cameras)
- Canon A620 (7 megapixels) with 4× optical zoom
- Nikon Coolpix S6 (6 megapixels)

It is important to remember that the higher the number of pixels, the greater is the "noise" created by the digital process. This noise cannot be easily removed by software manipulation. SLR digital cameras have the least noise, with Canon and Nikon finding excellent acceptance among phlebologists. "Point and shoot" digital cameras show the greatest noise, especially above 6–7 megapixels. The image stabilization facilities available with some camera systems will improve image quality.

Cameras that allow manual adjustment of white balance are to be preferred over those that only provide automatic white balance. All digital SLR cameras provide manual controls, while "point and shoot" cameras vary. Nikon provides lighting adjustments in the camera menus for immediate adjustment after the picture has been taken, which is very helpful. Sony cameras can also be adjusted, and tend to produce rich, overly saturated colors (especially red). Canon shows good light management, with colors that tend to be "soft", but very realistic.

Some cameras allow for magnification without the need for any additional hardware, including those produced by Panasonic, Nikon, Sony, and Canon. Magnification, without macro rings on the lenses, should be done with the camera's flash OFF. Macro rings are available for the Sony and Canon cameras (except for Canon's "point and shoot" series), but are unnecessary for the Nikon and Panasonic cameras.

Printer

Hewlett-Packard printers are frequently chosen, as their supplies are readily available and they currently have the widest variety of papers, including the standard for trifold brochures. However, the ink may be more expensive and require frequent replacement.

Canon printers are fast, their inks are more affordable, and other manufacturers' papers can be used. These printers also excel at double-sided printing and do not require attention during the process.

Epson and Lexmark (Dell) printers are a cost-effective option, but they are not as versatile or as durable if one has a high volume of printing.

Image storage and manipulation

Manipulation and storage of images are two activities that make digital photography especially useful to the practice of phlebology. With the correct software, it should be simple and take very little time to produce a good image at the time of each patient's visit.

Three popular programs for handling and working with photos are Adobe Photoshop, Microsoft Picture It, and Roxio Photosuite, while Kodak Easyshare and its Gallery may be used for cataloging the pictures. Some cameras come with their own photo-handling software, so an additional purchase is not necessary.

Portrait backdrops, slave flash lamps, macro rings, and reference distances can be obtained or made inexpensively, and can be used with all cameras. Digital pictures should be cataloged in a software management program and then burned onto CD-R discs for inclusion in the patient's chart and as a hard-copy backup. Selective hard-copy photographs for patient review or for insurance purposes are created from the CD. As treatment progresses in time, the CD may be used to easily show sequential improvement and is very economical in chart storage.

In conclusion, digital photography is fast and economical, and does not require advanced knowledge of computer graphics to master. It is an essential component of every phlebologist's office, and will greatly enhance both the practice and patients' understanding of improvements in their condition. It is best to have an area set up for taking photographs, with standardized background, distance, and lighting. These images are also useful for insurance documentation and for patient education.

Improving visualization: illumination and magnification

Proper examination and treatment require appropriate ambient illumination. Overhead fluorescent or focal fluorescent lights are the most common. A cold-light fiberoptic instrument (Venoscope, Vein-lite) as well as the newer infrared devices may be helpful in the local evaluation of varicose veins, as they improve the visibility of reticular veins. Examination tables should be chosen to allow the patient and phlebologist to be comfortable during the procedure. Mechanical tables have the advantage of allowing elevation or lowering of the patient's lower extremities in relation to the rest of the body – an important factor in enhancing the efficacy of treatment

In addition to illumination, telangiectasias may require magnification to fully appreciate feeding and tributary communication. It is best to try several magnification systems to determine which focal length, visual field width, and degree of magnification is preferred.

Sclerotherapy of large and small veins requires different needle calibers. A balance between patient comfort and safe injection technique must be struck. Needles of 30- to 33-gauge are usually used for injecting telangiectasias, 25-gauge needles are frequently used for procedures such as ultrasound- guided sclerotherapy, and 16- to 18-gauge needles are useful in removing trapped blood and for ambulatory phlebectomy. One should begin with small quantities of these products and find which perform the best in one's own office setting. Safety syringes in which the needle is withdrawn into the syringe following use and good technique with avoidance of recapping will diminish the incidence of needlesticks.

Syringes are made of single-use disposable plastic or sterilizable glass, and come with either a centrally or an eccentrically located hub. The latter places the needle closer to the skin for the shallow angle necessary for injection. The common syringe sizes are 5, 3, and 1 cm^3. Usually, 1 cm^3 syringes are used for more concentrated sclerosant doses for large veins, and 3–5 cm^3 syringes for telangiectasias, in which slow injection is preferable.

Endothermal ablative procedures require either radiofrequency (RF) or laser energy systems for the treatment of the truncal great saphenous or small saphenous veins. Investigation of these alternative procedures and the companies that provide the equipment is an important component in setting up a phlebology practice, as these procedures have demonstrated a superior outcome to surgery or sclerotherapy in many studies. Supply packs containing all the necessary components for the procedure are available from the equipment companies and many other vendors.

If the phlebologist performs surgical procedures, the appropriate instruments (hooks, etc.) are required in sufficient quantity for the number of cases performed, as is a sterilization system, which should be maintained and checked on a regular basis. If anesthesia is used during surgery, patient monitoring and resuscitation devices and supplies are also required.

In the United States, sclerosants are currently obtained from pharmaceutical companies and compounding pharmacies. The

phlebologist should be familiar with the dilution and side-effects of each medication used. Detergent sclerosing agents can be agitated with air or carbon dioxide to produce foam, which has advantages over a liquid sclerosant. Emergency medications and equipment should be on hand in case of severe allergic reactions or other serious complications.

External compression is a mainstay of primary therapy in phlebology practice, and is frequently used following all phlebological procedures. Various forms of compression, such as low-stretch bandages, Unna's boot, and graduated compression elastic stockings should be available in the office. Application of external compression should only be carried out after assessing the peripheral arterial circulation. Relationships with manufacturers' sales representatives are helpful in order to obtain information on new products and to keep a working supply of compression stockings available for patients.

Several products are available to aid in the placement of the stocking. A nylon foot sleeve comes with each stocking to ease the stocking over the toes. Rubber gloves help the patient to grip the stocking. There are also zippered stockings, as well as a device known as a "butler" (Medi USA, LP, Whitsett, NC). The "butler" expands the stocking over a metal frame, allowing for easier foot insertion, coupled with handgrips to advance the stocking proximally. Metal rings are available to stretch the stocking in order to easily place it over the pads that are sometimes used after sclerotherapy. A two-layered sleeve made of nylon material is also available (Easy-Slide by BSN-JOBST, Inc., Charlotte, NC) that assists patients in donning an open-toed stocking.

If the practice is broad, including leg swelling and ulceration, competence must be gained in application of below-the-knee dressings, including low-stretch bandages or Unna's boot. Foam pads are utilized to provide increased local compression over incompetent perforating veins and around the malleoli. Foam pads can be cut from sheets of high-density foam rubber or are commercially available in precut shapes.

Surgical treatment of varicose veins may require general, regional, or local anesthesia. Sclerotherapy generally does not require anesthesia, although some patients benefit from oral anxiolytics or the topical application of anesthetic ointments or creams. Because of the ambulatory nature of sclerotherapy and the potential for thrombosis, it is wise to keep the patient as active as possible.

During the consultation with the patient, the findings of the physical examination, treatment options, and treatment plans are discussed. Prior to any procedure, the patient must have a general understanding of the procedure, including the benefit of treatment, and its risks, alternatives, and side-effects, as well as the risks of not having the treatment. A consent form, signed by the patient and physician, provides a vehicle for a frank discussion, allowing questions to be fully answered before treatment.

Each patient begins the process by stating "I don't expect perfection," but experience indicates that many do. This is an important time to establish realistic expectations in the mind of the patient. Along with a good physician–patient relationship, this will result in an increased level of trust and satisfaction for both the physician and the patient. Since superficial venous disease is known to be chronic and progressive, it is wise to stress the palliative nature of all treatment and the high likelihood that progression may warrant additional treatment in the future.

Insurance

Geographic location and type of practice (surgery, sclerotherapy, and/or laser) will result in various levels of insurance reimbursement. In general, coverage is usually limited to large varicose veins (especially those associated with pain that is unrelieved by conservative measures), edema, pre-ulcerative skin changes, phlebitis, hemorrhage, or ulceration. Most treatment for telangiectasias is considered cosmetic.

Malpractice coverage needs to be obtained for all treatment modalities. Documentation of the discussion of the risks, benefits, alternatives, and the procedures, as well as pretreatment photographs, are important factors in risk management.

Promotion

Building a phlebology practice takes time, patient referrals, physician referrals, and long-term good results. Methods to let the public know how to find the practice include educational seminars, public relations, and advertising. It is wise to develop a patient brochure, as this provides take-home information for each patient. Brochures are available in a ready-made format free of charge from the Federal Trade Commission; the American College of Phlebology has also produced a very informative brochure. Customized or practice-specific brochures can be especially helpful, as they provide patients and prospective patients with an introduction to venous disease, the practice philosophy, and specifics about the office. Increasing use of the Internet by patients may encourage the development of a practice website.

Local radio and TV stations always need spokespersons to answer questions about vein treatment. Advertising on radio or television are options that require careful preparation and a large outlay of capital, but may be helpful in introducing a new base of prospective patients to the practice.

Conclusion

Starting a phlebology practice can be a daunting task. A thorough understanding of venous disease and the various treatment options must precede the opening of any practice. It is wise for the phlebologist to continue to obtain didactic and hands-on training, since this field is developing rapidly and techniques are improving faster than the literature can keep up with. Patients are usually extremely grateful for expert evaluation of venous complaints, and treatment outcomes are generally very gratifying for both patient and physician.

Bibliography

Browse NL, Burnand KG, Irvine AT, Wilson NM, eds. Diseases of the Veins, 2nd edn. London: Arnold, 1999.

Gloviczki P, Yao JST, eds. Handbook of Venous Disorders, 2nd edn. New York: Arnold, 2001.

Goldman MP, Bergan JL, Guex JJ. Sclerotherapy: Treatment of Varicose and Telangiectatic Leg Veins, 4th edn. St Louis, MO: Mosby, 2007.

Sadick NS. Manual of Sclerotherapy. Philadelphia: Lippincott Williams and Wilkins, 2000.

Schadeck M. Duplex Phlebology. Naples: Gnocchi, 1994.

Tretbar LL. Venous Disorders of the Legs – Principles and Practice. London: Springer-Verlag, 1999.

Venous Digest. http://www.venousdigest.com.

Weiss RA, Feied CF, Weiss MA. Vein Diagnosis and Treatment: A Comprehensive Approach. New York: McGraw-Hill, 2001.

The American College of Phlebology (ACP) was formed and incorporated in 1986 as the North American Society of Phlebology. Twelve years later, in order to better reflect our educational purpose, the society's name was changed to the American College of Phlebology. As set out by our visionary founders, the ACP has always been an inclusive organization. The College has taken a broad approach to the advancement of the field, welcomes physicians from various specialty backgrounds, and recognizes nurses and ultrasonographers as valued contributors. In this way, knowledge is disseminated, greater insights realized, and the care of a vast group of patients improved more rapidly.

The history of the College has been one of dramatic growth and expansion. Our first Annual Scientific Congress was held in San Diego in February 1988. Since then, we have held regional symposia and a scientific congress each year. Our Annual Congress includes separate symposia organized by the Phlebology Nursing Section and by the Ultrasonography Section. In 2007 ACP meetings brought nearly a thousand physicians and allied healthcare providers together to hear the latest in scientific advances in the field of phlebology and to learn from a variety of keynote lectures, small group sessions, instructional courses, and hands-on workshops. As of this book's publication date, we have over 1700 physician and allied health members, and we continue to grow.

In meeting the challenge of educating its diverse membership, the Board commissioned a survey in June of 2005 to identify the most critical priorities. The results focused the Board's efforts on specialty recognition, board certification, academic fellowship programs, expanded educational meetings, and research interests.

As a result of the initiatives undertaken by the ACP the American Medical Association (AMA) approved the College's application for recognition of phlebology as a self-designated practice specialty. This recognition is a pivotal step toward increasing the credibility and visibility of the specialty to colleagues in other fields, industry, and patients. Recently, the American Osteopathic Association also recognized phlebology as a distinct practice discipline, as have a number of state medical organizations.

The ACP Board recognized the opportunity and responsibility that came with the AMA decision, but realized that the initiatives our membership wanted required the commitment of major resources. To secure such resources, the American College of Phlebology Foundation (ACPF) was launched at our November 2006 Annual Congress. These major achievements laid the groundwork for the expansion of programs and initiatives, for this year and well into our future.

Strategically, defining the content of phlebology training programs became the next priority. The ACP published its first statement regarding content in its official journal, *Phlebology*. Following this, the ACP Board Certification Development Task Force selected an outside organization to assist in the development of a comprehensive, high-quality, psychometrically valid exam in phlebology. In support and partnership with ACP the ACPF Board approved funding the development of the exam. The first American Board of Phlebology Certification exam will be offered in April 2008. The 200-item computer-based exam will be delivered in over 4000 authorized test centers worldwide. The ACP Board announced the creation of a Phlebology Fellowship, patterned after an Accreditation Council for Graduate Medical Education (ACGME) postgraduate medical training program and defined by The Fellowship Program Committee, that provides 12 months of postgraduate training in phlebology. After a competitive selection process, the first ACP Phlebology Fellowship program was approved at the University of California San Diego under the direction of Dr John J Bergan and commenced in July 2007. Graduates of approved Phlebology Fellowships will be eligible to sit for the Board Certification in Phlebology. Applications to host a Phlebology Fellowship in the United States are available on the ACP website (http://www.phlebology.org).

The ACP also offers various research grant programs. Three grants, with an annual amount of up to $150 000, are funded by the ACP Foundation. The grants have varied audiences: junior faculty investigators with a career interest in phlebology research, clinical phlebologists, as well as young investigators still in medical school and not yet professionally established in the phlebological sciences. Another phlebology grant offered by the ACP annually is for $15 000 and is underwritten by Jobst, a subsidiary of BSN Medical. All grant applications are available on the ACP website. The Research Programs Committee strives to ensure that projects are distributed over a range of topics representative of the breadth and diversity of the field of phlebology.

The American College of Phlebology is poised to have an enormous impact on the care of patients with venous disease. We continue to seek new opportunities to improve the education of physicians, medical staff, and laypersons about phlebology and to advance the highest standard of care for patients with venous disease. The College welcomes new members, and offers training, continuing education and networking opportunities for your entire office staff. For more information or to receive a membership application, please visit the ACP website or contact the American College of Phlebology at +1 (510) 834-6500.

Reference

1. Nguyen T, Bergan J, Min R, Morrison N, Zimmet S. Curriculum of the American College of Phlebology. Phlebology 2006; 21(Suppl 2): 1–20.